POWER BODY

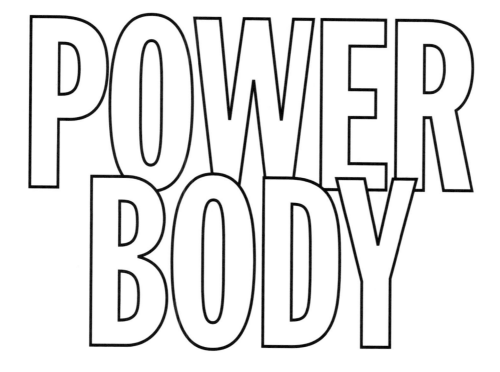

POWER BODY

Tom Seabourne, Ph.D.

YMAA Publication Center
Boston, Mass. USA

YMAA Publication Center
Main Office:
  4354 Washington Street
  Boston, Massachusetts, 02131
  617-323-7215 • ymaa@aol.com • www.ymaa.com

10 9 8 7 6 5 4 3 2 1

Edited by James O'Leary
Cover Design by Richard Rossiter

ISBN:1-886969-76-0

Anatomy drawings copyright ©1994 by TechPool Studios Corp. USA, 1463 Warrensville
Center Road, Cleveland, OH 44121

Publisher's Cataloging in Publication
(Prepared by Quality Books Inc.)

Seabourne, Thomas.
    Power Body : injury prevention, rehabilitation
and sports performance enhancement / Tom
Seabourne. – 1st ed.
    p. cm.
    LCCN: 99-
    ISBN: 1-886969-76-0

    1. Sports injuries—Prevention—Popular works.
2. Martial arts—Training. 3. Sports medicine—
Popular works. I. Title.

RD97.S43 1999   617.1'027
                                  QBI99-799

Disclaimer:
The authors and publisher of this material are NOT RESPONSIBLE in any manner
whatsoever for any injury which may occur through reading or following the instructions
in this manual.
The activities, physical or otherwise, described in this material may be too strenuous or
dangerous for some people, and the reader(s) should consult a physician before engaging
in them.

Printed in Canada

Foreword

Over the years we at Topper Sportsmedicine in Vail, Colorado have had the opportunity to work with the best athletes in the world. Professional tennis players like Monica Seles, football player John Elway, and many others, put their trust in us to get them back out on the court or field in record time.

My life has been helping people to become their best. Every day I meet patients with knee, back, shoulder, foot, and elbow problems. They want to be cured, right now. Our job is to help them achieve their goal, and in the process teach them about their bodies in order to minimize their chances for a return visit.

To this end, we have designed a variety of exercises and pieces of equipment. Many of them presented in this book, and in conjunction with the concepts presented here, we feel they can help rehabilitate and actually improve performance in your numerous sports or activities.

Power Body is a book that should serve as an easy reference whenever you need to rehabilitate or condition yourself for your favorite form of exercise. Whatever sports you enjoy, *Power Body* will help you play them better, faster, harder, and longer.

Power Body teaches you to speed your metabolism, gain muscle, lose fat, and stay healthy. Other things you will learn in this book include:

- Training techniques to improve your sports performance.
- The best and worst fitness equipment.
- Specific instruction required to rehabilitate and condition yourself.
- The risks and injuries associated with your sport.
- Prevention and treatment of your sports related injuries.

The method is simple. Choose your favorite section of *Power Body*. Begin reading. But set your alarm to buzz at twenty-minute intervals. No matter how engrossed you are, stand up for two minutes between every twenty-minute reading session, and physically perform one of the exercises you just read about. Then sit yourself back down and flip through more pages until another topic excites you. Repeat this cycle until your brain is full and your physique is awesome. Your motivation for healthy living begins here.

Topper Hagerman, Ph.D
Topper Sportsmedicine
Vail, Colorado
June 29, 1999

Preface

Power Body introduces you to the precarious nature of your martial art. I teach you how to practice anywhere, anytime, and anyplace.

Simple, step-by-step drills, exercises, and techniques will provide you with THE EDGE. If you use my strategies to become stronger, faster, and have more coordination, endurance, and flexibility than your opponent, you will probably win.

A side-benefit of martial arts is improved body composition. Body composition is your muscle to fat ratio. You can accelerate your fat loss and muscle gain by knowing a little about eating. Unlike dieting, I make eating fun. You will learn how to eat to fuel your muscle and starve your fat cells. This speeds your metabolism for increased energy and improved martial arts performance.

Mind/body strategies will benefit you as a child, adult, or grandparent. You will learn how to relax, focus, and be your best in any martial arts situation you can imagine.

Maybe you never thought of yourself as a physiologist or diagnostician. But *Power Body* helps you to recognize common martial arts injuries and how to treat them. You will learn just enough about anatomy and first aid so you won't be confused. You will amaze your martial arts instructor with your knowledge about the shoulder, knee, back, and abs.

Have you harbored a secret desire to phone the American Red Cross, to find out the percentage of heart attack victims who are actually revived by CPR? Or would you be curious to know what percent fat you're allowed to eat on the Pritikin diet? The bad news is, that the answer to both of these questions is roughly fifteen percent.

Acknowledgements

Thanks to the unwavering support of my wife, Danese, and my children Alaina, Grant, Laura, Susanna, and Julia. To my mother, Ann Seabourne, my brother, Rick, and my sister, Barbara who held our lives together during the unexpected passing of my father who was the inspiration for this book. Thanks also to Bruce Crawford for his help with the photographs.

Introduction

If you're like many martial artists, you have a nagging hip, foot, shoulder, or knee injury that just won't heal. But you love your martial arts training, and the "rest" that your doctor ordered is not an option.

Face it, injury happens, no matter how careful you are. My goal with *Power Body* is to keep you in your game. What if you could recognize your strain, sprain, or fracture, and use my secrets to heal faster and stronger?

Power Body teaches you to speed your metabolism, gain muscle, lose fat, and stay healthy. Other things you will learn in this book include:

- Training techniques to improve your martial arts performance.
- The risks and injuries associated with your sport.
- Prevention and treatment of your sports related injuries.

How to use this book. There are many ways to use this book. Scan a few pages here and there. Read it from A to Z. Or even memorize and recite the entire text aloud.

- **Cover-To-Cover:** Read every page of *Power Body* and you will find yourself to be the most popular martial artist in your neighborhood. Newfound buddies will ask you to treat their plantar fasciitis. Or they will quiz you on the pros and cons of whether they should wear a knee brace. Be careful. Although your brain will be as full as a medical encyclopedia, for liability reasons, always suggest your friends consult their physicians before using your exercise prescription.

- **Read What You Need:** Do you run low on energy from time to time? Has it become a routine to visit your doctor for your quarterly B-12 injection? Before contributing to your HMO, try thumbing through my book first.

  It may seem easier for your doctor to inject a magic bullet (even if it is just a placebo). But I think it might be more fun for you to follow my tried-and-true, non-pharmaceutical, energy boosting strategies.

- **Follow ALL of the steps:** Just as your doctor required you to finish your entire antibiotic prescription, please follow my step-by-step injury prevention, exercise, and eating plans to their conclusion. Give my programs a fair chance. If you quit too soon, you may miss incredible benefits. Besides, I want you to be so pleased with your progress, that you recommend this book to everyone you meet.

- **Use common sense:** Although this book is for every martial artist, your particular body type or disposition may not allow you to enjoy EVERY SINGLE STRATEGY presented in *Power Body*. I have never seen a training program or book I fully agreed with. And I don't expect you to fully agree with me about everything. Just use what works for you and ignore the rest.

How This Book Is Organized. This book has several different sections, and an appendices. Feel free to pinball from part to part at your leisure. No section depends on another. If you are interested in knee problems, you may shy away from the stretching section. But I hope you don't. You might be surprised to discover that if you improve your hamstring flexibility, your knees may heal sooner. And relaxed muscles help you to be more confident in the dojo.

CHAPTER ONE

Balance In Your Training

Living Well

Martial artists are balanced. They get up when they get knocked down. Their training is a juggling act between their mental, spiritual, social, and emotional lives.

Martial artists train for health, fitness, and skill development.

Exercising for health is as simple as a twenty-minute kata and sparring session at a vigorous pace three or four times a week. Two thirty-minute strength training sessions are a "healthy" workout. A five-minute warm-up and cool-down is included.

Fitness training is a little more vigorous than twenty minutes of exercise three times a week. Martial artists who train for fitness work their cardiovascular systems forty minutes, four or five times per week, by kicking and punching using moderate intensity. And they strength train by splitting their body parts to work different muscle groups on different days. They also perform an appropriate warm-up and cool-down.

Martial arts skill development training is specific to your goals. Self-defense, sparring, kata, grappling, and mind/body unity are worthwhile pursuits.

Balanced martial artists utilize a combination of health, fitness, and skill development strategies. Unlike marathoners who have trouble carrying a heavy suitcase, weight lifters who huff and puff climbing a flight of stairs, or bodybuilders who have difficulty combing their hair, martial artists enjoy diversity in their training.

You can choose to improve your health, fitness, and martial arts skills, or you can remain on the couch. Eating marbled steak and fried potatoes might sound better than a chicken breast sandwich, at first. Lounging through a sitcom seems more appealing than practicing forms. But after awhile, your body requires action.

Goal Setting

Success in any endeavor is measured in achievement. Reaching lofty goals seems easy for some—until we peer behind the scenes. Consider doctors, lawyers, and professional athletes. We sometimes forget how hard they worked in the classroom or on the playing field. Some paid an awesome toll early, and later reaped tremendous rewards.

You too have the opportunity to experience martial arts beyond your wildest expectations. And you can enjoy the process. But first you must prepare. Close your eyes and take a few moments to determine your desires. Don't hesitate to explore seemingly unattainable ideals. Make a detailed wishlist. Nothing is far-fetched. Fantasize for hours, days, months. It takes as long as it takes. Make mental notes or write them down. How would it feel to be participating in martial arts? Attain mastery with your heart and mind. Feel victorious from the tips of your toes to the top of your head.

Next, set achievable short-term goals that will equip you to tackle your mission. This may require research. Locate a studio. Choose some exercises from this book. Begin training. Early achievements serve as motivation. Daily short-term targets inspire you. Small successes provide endurance for the long haul.

No worthwhile goal is simple. Prepare for distractions and obstacles. Motivation will wax and wane and there will be pitfalls. Stay focused. Be careful of those who may sabotage your efforts. Part of your duties may be unrelated to your chosen dream. You may embrace martial arts competitions but detest hours of training. Sometimes you are required to bide your time when you prefer action.

While focusing on martial arts you may perceive yourself as one-dimensional. Keep your options open. Strive to be well rounded. Have it all but guard your priorities. Make daily choices based on your priorities, then your mission. Fall asleep at a reasonable hour and awaken early to prepare your day. Each hour brings you closer to your health, fitness, and martial arts goal. And don't forsake friends. Cherish God and your family. In the end they matter most.

Winning or losing does not affect your progress. If you are disappointed with an outcome search to discover how you may improve. Each martial arts workout provides you with the information to be better next time. Constructive criticism provides insight. Improvement doesn't come fast or easy. Sometimes a breakthrough takes years of disciplined training. But let go and relax. If you try too hard you undermine your efforts. Ask yourself, "Why am I training?" Think about the reasons you began.

Opportunities to rise to the next level are scarce. Be on the lookout for a break. Read. Write letters to establish rapport with possible mentors. Keep an eye out for seminars that relate to your dream. You may receive a phone call to attend a martial arts camp. Or a sensei may mysteriously find you. Although you are busy in your wearisome grind, pay attention to these magic moments.

Success is not just being better than someone else is. It's what you do outside of your striving that counts. There are thousands who reach martial arts success and would gladly trade it for inner peace. Taking giant steps over your competition is addicting and sometimes abusive. Self-gratification and high achievement alone is not the answer. Rather than treading on folks, carry them. Give yourself permission to be your best and help your comrades along the way. Emptiness is at the top unless you support your friends. It is not about winning and losing but reaching your potential. Anybody can struggle to become a martial arts champion, but how many toil to help others become one?

Training in the Year 2000

Martial artists are in search of the illusive six-pack. Sit-ups have been replaced with crunches. Rather than frenetically bouncing up and down, the crunch is smooth and measured. Try it. Lie on your back with your arms to your sides. Set a metronome at forty beats per minute (BPM), or hum one-one-thousand, two-one-thousand, etc. for each crunch. Lift your rib cage towards your pubis moving your fingers three inches for each repetition (Figure 1-1).

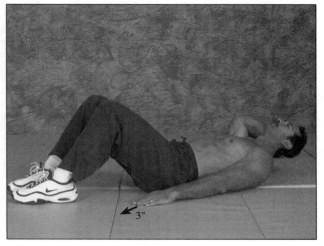

Figure 1-1

Perform as many crunches as possible, but there is no hurry as you are required to stay with the beat. You are not permitted to rest in either the up or down position. Fifty crunches is an outstanding score for women, and sixty is excellent for men. You should finish with no neck or back pain. The crunch is a more valid and a much safer appraisal of abdominal muscular endurance than sit-ups.

Almost all serious martial artists participate in some form of resistance training. Weight training should be performed according to new ACSM regulations:

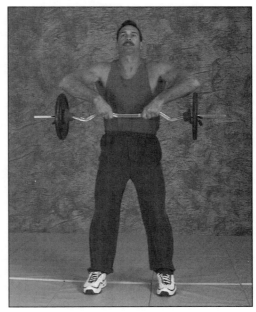

Figure 1-2

- Upright rows for your trapezius: Raise the weight no higher than sixty degrees to avoid stress on the shoulder (Figures 1-2 to 1-4).

- Supine (on your back) chest flyes for your pectorals: Do not let your elbows break the frontal plane (go below parallel) to avoid stress on the static stabilizers of the shoulder (ligaments and connective tissue) as well as the dynamic stabilizers (rotator cuff muscles) (Figures 1-5 to 1-7).

- Behind the neck lat pull downs for your latissimus dorsi: Your shoulders are at a high risk for injury when your arms are abducted (pulled away from your body) and externally rotated (pulled back) as in the behind the neck lat pull down (Figures 1-8 and

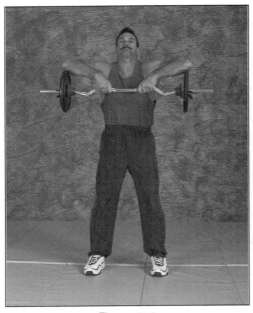

Figure 1-3

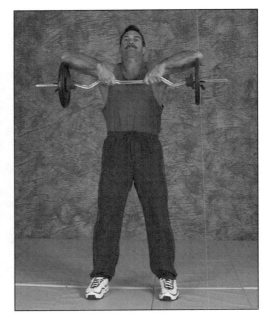

Figure 1-4

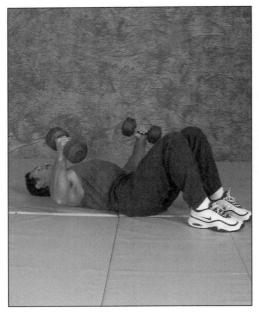

Figure 1-5

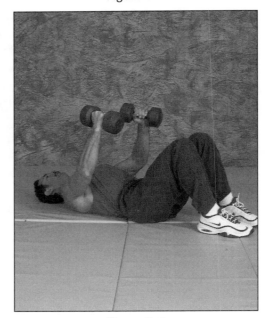

Figure 1-6

1-9). The front pull down is much safer with no sacrifice to muscle involvement. The front pull down also avoids the possibility of damage to your cervical vertebrae.

- Squats and lunges for your quadriceps and hamstrings: The risk is to your knees if you squat below ninety degrees, if your toes are not aligned with your knees, or if the weight you are lifting is too heavy (Figures 1-10 to 1-15).

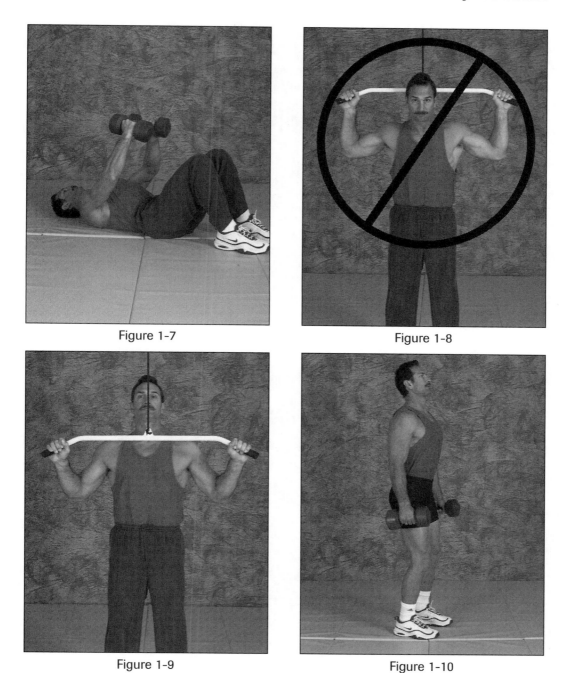

Figure 1-7

Figure 1-8

Figure 1-9

Figure 1-10

The jury is still out concerning nutritional supplementation. Many new products are untested over the long term. There are no federal controls over some of these substances. You are never sure what you are paying for. And the amount or purity of these products may be suspect. Replacing foods with supplements might cause you to miss out on different vitamins,

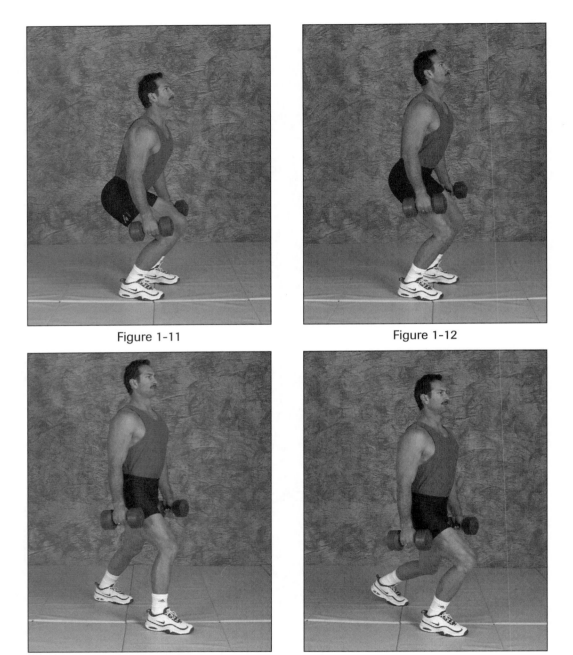

Figure 1-11

Figure 1-12

Figure 1-13

Figure 1-14

minerals, and fibers. In addition, taking increased dosages could inhibit the absorption of other important nutrients.

Recently it was found that shorter, more frequent martial arts workouts can be more beneficial than longer programs, for certain populations. Beginners, the very deconditioned, and those with disease, require several, condensed sessions. Some folks are simply incapable of maintaining a longer routine. The number of calories burned is dependent on the amount of work performed, regardless of whether it was continuous or intermittent. Improvement in the cardiovascular system is dependent on continuity (minimum of fifteen minutes), however. Therefore, brief bouts of martial arts can offer skill and health benefits, but not necessarily fitness improvements.

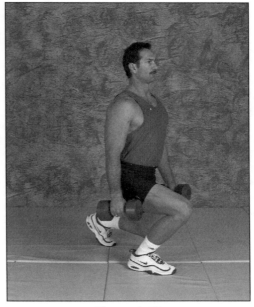

Figure 1-15

Flexibility

Stretching is a relaxing way to finish your workout. Improving your flexibility increases your range of motion and circulation. Stretching also decreases your injury potential and aids in healing.

Stretch slow and steady to avoid the stretch reflex. The stretch reflex occurs when your muscles tighten to avoid being stretched too fast or too far. You can override the stretch reflex by relaxing into your stretch instead of bouncing.

Specific rewards of stretching include improved martial arts skills, recovery time, coordination, balance, reaction time, quickness, and decreased injury potential.

Pre-Post Fitness Testing: Strengths And Weaknesses. The purpose of fitness testing for you as a martial artist is to determine strengths and weaknesses in your program. Heart rate measures help to determine your recovery rate. It's nice to know your body fat so you can adjust your eating to your martial arts programming. Muscular strength and endurance can be assessed with the crunch, bench press, and push-up tests. You can improve your muscular endurance by practicing the test exercises themselves. And you will probably score in the upper ranges of flexibility if you perform the minimum stretches required of a martial artist.

- Heart Rate Evaluation: The purpose is to measure frequency of your heart's contractions. It is measured in beats per minute (BPM).

    Measure your heart rate by placing your fingertips on a pulse site such as your carotid artery or inside your wrist. If you have a stethoscope, position the bell on the third intercostal space to the left of your sternum (Figures 1-16 and 1-17).

    Heart rate watches and monitors consist of a chest strap containing electrodes that register your heartbeat. These devices cost between $150 and $300.

    Heart rates range from 40 to 100 BPM. The average for men is 70 BPM. Women average 75 BPM. Elite martial artists generally have lower resting heart rates, but not always.

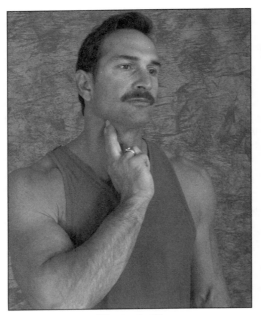
Figure 1-16

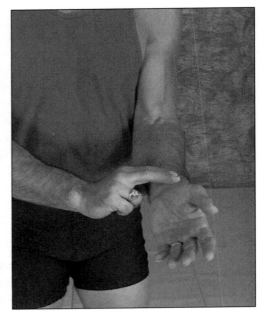
Figure 1-17

Resting heart rate is most accurately measured before rising from your bed in the morning. During the day, be seated fifteen minutes prior to taking your count.

Your pulse should be taken for sixty seconds. Or, take it for thirty seconds and double the number. Exercise heart rate should be taken for six seconds so you may return to your martial arts. Multiply your total by ten. The product is your exercise BPM.

- Body Composition Evaluation: The purpose for measuring your body composition is to determine your percent body fat in comparison to your total body weight. Excess body fat is a secondary risk factor for coronary artery disease (CAD).

Hydrostatic weighing is considered the "gold standard" for measuring body fat. Your body density is calculated from the relationship between your normal body weight and your underwater weight. Fat weighs less than water.

Bioelectrical impedance measures your body fat by passing an electric current from your finger to your toe. The conductivity of an electrical impulse is faster through lean tissue than through fat. You should be well hydrated, not have practiced martial arts within six hours, and consumed no alcohol twenty-four hours before the test, for an accurate reading.

Skinfold measurements are based on the presumption that fifty percent of your total body fat is just below your skin. The experimenter pinches three sites on your body. For men these include your chest, abdomen and thigh. The average percent body fat for men is twelve to eighteen percent. For women the sites are your triceps, suprailliac, and thigh. Women average between eighteen and twenty-five percent body fat.

- Waist to Hip Ratio Evaluation: The more weight you carry in your belly, the higher your risk for CAD. Use a tape measure to assess your waist and hips in inches. Divide your waist by your hip measurement.

  If your waist is thirty-six inches and your hips are forty-two inches (36/42 = 0.85), this signifies a moderate/high risk for CAD. High CAD risk for men is greater than 1.0. For women, high risk is greater than 0.85.

- Push-up Test: The purpose of the push-up test is to measure muscular endurance. Perform as many push-ups as possible. Do not rest in either the up or down position.

  Men assume the standard push-up position with their knees straight. Hands are shoulder width apart. Chests come three inches from the floor with each repetition.

  Women rest their knees on the floor. An excellent score for men is over fifty push-ups. For women, thirty is an excellent score.

- Bench Press Test: This is another muscular endurance test. The weight is set at eighty pounds. Lie on a flat bench. A metronome is set at 60 BPM. Spotters are present for safety.

  Repetitions are counted when your elbows are fully extended (not locked), and the bar comes down to your chest. The test is concluded when you cannot maintain form, or lose the beat of the metronome.

  An excellent score for men is thirty-seven repetitions. For women the test is identical except the weight is set at thirty-five pounds. An excellent score for women is thirty-five repetitions.

- Canadian Crunch Test: The purpose of this test is to measure muscular endurance of your abdominal area. Lie on your back with your arms extended to your sides. Place a strip of tape on the floor at the end of your fingertips. Place another piece of tape three inches away from the first strip.

  To perform a proper crunch, curl your rib cage toward your pelvis. Your fingers move from one strip of tape to the next. Perform as many crunches as possible to a 40 BPM metronome setting.

  The test is completed when you cannot execute another crunch. An excellent score for men is sixty. Women receive an outstanding score after performing fifty repetitions.

- Trunk Flexion Test: The purpose of the trunk flexion test is to measure flexibility of your lower back and hamstrings. Take your shoes off and sit with your knees straight and your feet twelve inches apart. Place a yardstick between your legs with the fifteen inch mark even with your feet. The zero inch mark should be closer to your knees.

  Place one of your hands on top of the other. The tips of your fingers are aligned. Exhale and slowly lean forward by dropping your head toward your arms. Your fingers slide over the yardstick (Figures 1-18 to 1-19).

  Take the best of three measurements. An excellent score for men is greater than twenty inches. A superior grade for women is more than twenty-four inches.

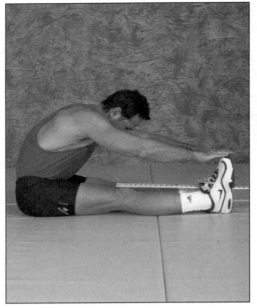

Figure 1-18

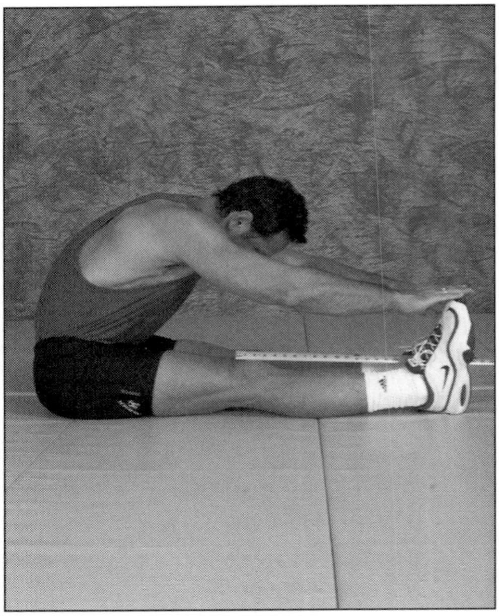

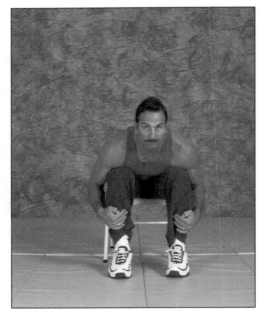

Figure 1-19

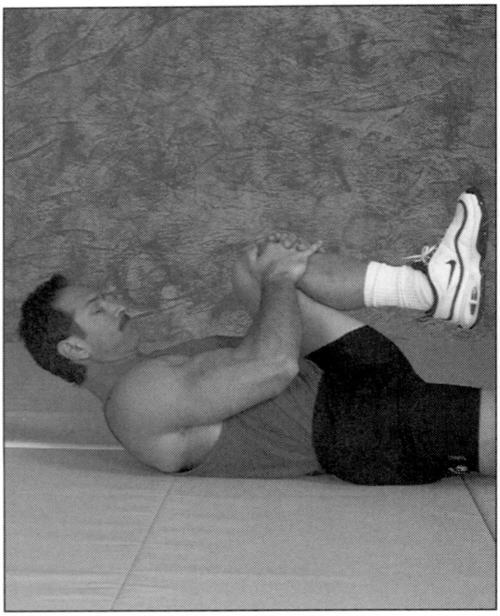

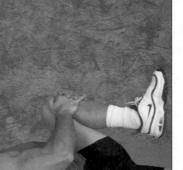

Figure 1-20

Figure 1-21

- Hip Flexion Test: The purpose of the hip flexion test is to determine if your hip flexors (the muscles that lift your knees) are too tight. Lie on your back. Maintain a flat lower back while grabbing behind your left knee. Pull your left knee to your chest (Figure 1-20).

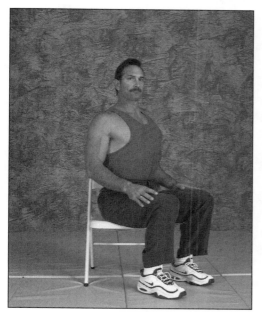

Figure 1-22

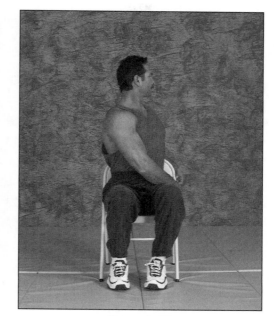

Figure 1-23

Normal flexibility is indicated when your right leg remains flat on the floor. Your hip flexors are considered tight if you attempt to lift your left knee toward your chest, and your right leg leaves the floor. Repeat with your other leg.

Injury Prevention: Flexibility Training. If you find yourself in the same position for extended periods, try stretching in the opposite direction. Stretch your lower back (quadratus laborum, erector spinae) by leaning forward in your chair, using your arms for support, and place your chest on your thighs (Figure 1-21).

Then press yourself into an upright position and pull your shoulders back (scapular retraction) to stretch your chest (pectorals) (Figure 1-22).

Stretch the sides of your trunk (obliques)

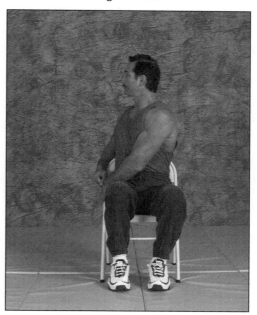

Figure 1-24

by twisting slowly to one side and then the other (Figures 1-23 and 1-24).

Rest your ankle on your thigh into a figure-4 position. Lean your chest toward your knee, stretching your hip (gluteus and piriformis). Switch legs and repeat (Figures 1-25 and 1-26).

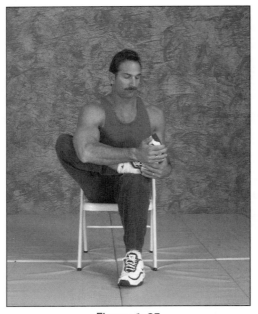

Figure 1-25

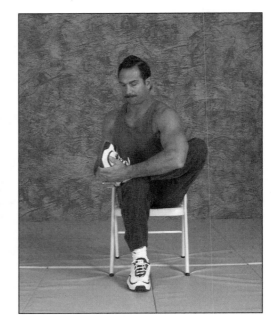

Figure 1-26

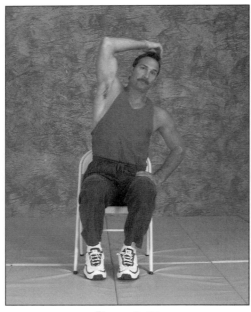

Figure 1-27

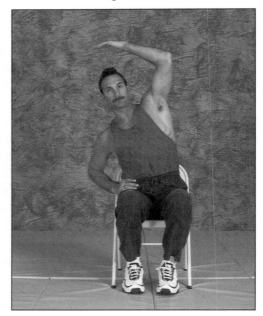

Figure 1-28

Raise one arm above your head and place the other hand on your hip. Lean sideways until you feel a stretch in your waist. Switch hands and repeat (Figures 1-27 and 1-28).

Grab your right elbow with your left hand and pull it as high as you can stretching the back of your arm (triceps) and upper back (latissimus dorsi). Switch arms and repeat (Figures 1-29 and 1-30).

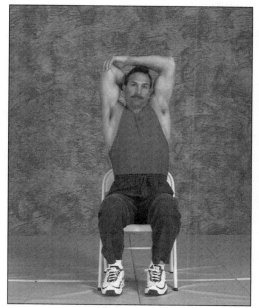

Figure 1-29

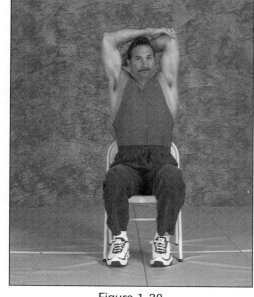

Figure 1-30

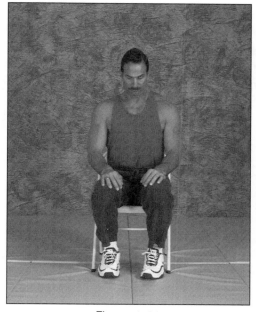

Figure 1-31

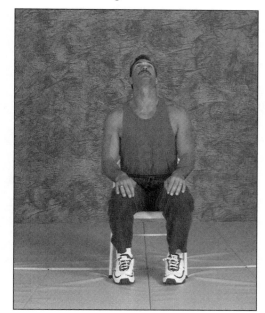

Figure 1-32

Stretch your neck and trapezius muscles by bringing your chin to your chest. Then slowly look toward the ceiling. Bring your right ear toward your right shoulder and your left ear toward your left shoulder (Figures 1-31 to 1-34).

Stretch after you warm up and before vigorous martial arts training.

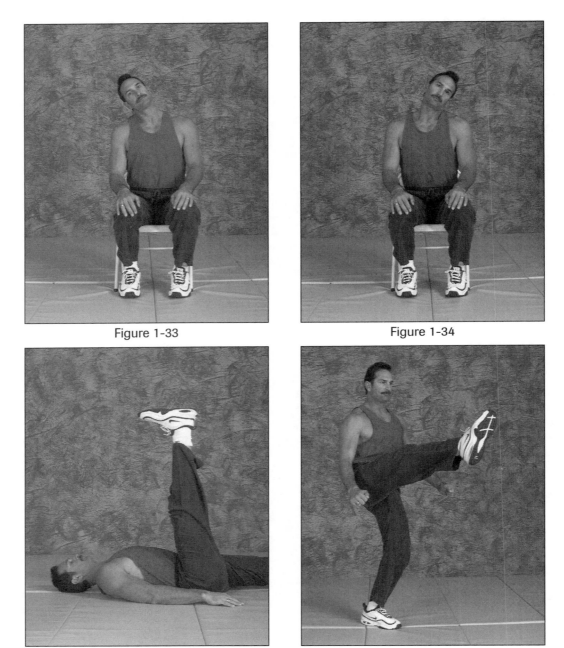

Figure 1-33

Figure 1-34

Figure 1-35

Figure 1-36

Performance Improvement: Dynamic Stretching. Let's try an experiment. You be the subject. Lie on your back. Keep both knees just slightly bent and raise your right leg up toward the ceiling until you feel a stretch in your hamstring (Figure 1-35). Hold that stretch and take note of the angle of your leg in reference to your body.

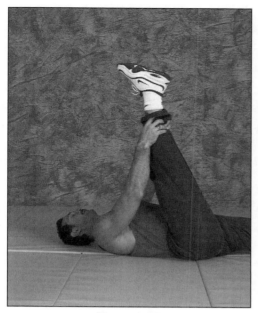

Figure 1-37

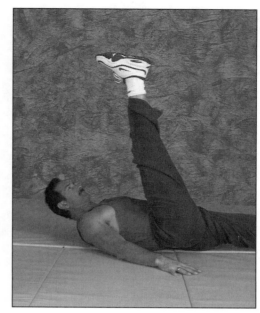

Figure 1-38

Now stand. Raise your right leg up again (Figure 1-36). How far did you lift it before your leg stopped going up? What angle was your leg at your peak stretch? Why couldn't you raise you leg to the same degree as when you were lying on the floor?

Try another experiment. Lie on your back and raise your leg as you did before (Figure 1-37). This time, grab your ankle and slowly add a few inches to your previous stretch until you feel slight discomfort in your hamstrings.

Release your grip and attempt to hold your leg in your newfound extended stretch (Figure 1-38). If your leg did what mine did when I performed this experiment, it bounced back down about thirty degrees.

Our goal is to eliminate that thirty degree drop. Obviously, our hamstrings were flexible enough to extend that extra thirty degrees in the first place, but we needed help to pull our leg into position. Why couldn't we continue to hold our leg in the extended stretch when we released our grip?

The answer to this question is, and you may or may not believe it when you look into a mirror, but we are just not strong enough. The reason your leg dropped thirty degrees was a lack of muscle strength and stability. The antagonist muscles to your hamstrings are your quadriceps and hip flexors. These muscles must be extremely strong to hold your hamstrings in a lengthened stretch.

Here's the point. It is wonderful to amaze your friends with hyper-flexibility, performing Chinese splits and front splits on the floor, but does floor flexibility translate into effective kicking?

I have developed a new stretching program to increase dynamic flexibility. That is, your ability to kick higher. This exciting strategy is simple, pain free, and easy to follow. It is tried-and-true, and passes muster with contemporary fitness gurus.

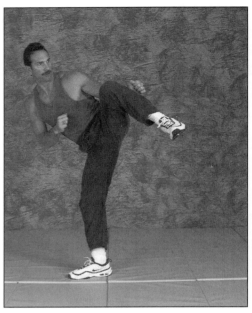

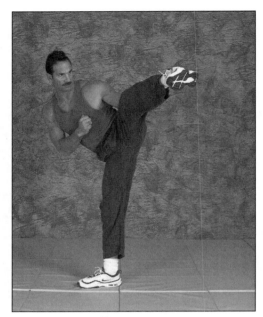

Figure 1-39   Figure 1-40

Please follow the steps below. Your training hall should be quiet and calm. The temperature should be warm, no less than eighty degrees Fahrenheit.

Take your time through all of the procedures; do not rush these exercises. Make this stretching sequence predictable so that your body *knows* what to do next and your mind can *focus* on your stretch. Be mindful of your muscles throughout each and every exercise to achieve your best stretch. Breathe calmly at the edge of discomfort as you execute each stretch/kick and swing. Realize that your stretch *will* improve and that this IS the perfect stretch for you *today.*

- Ten Minutes of Shadow Boxing: Begin facing a mirror in a sparring stance. Throw slow and low, front kicks. One with each leg. Then alternate slow-low roundhouse kicks. And finally slow-low side kicks with each leg. Mix easy punches into your kicks as if you were shadow sparring. Gradually increase the height of each kick. Kick slow and controlled. Keep your upper body relaxed and in perfect sparring position. As your body warms up, kick higher and higher. Continue to alternate legs. Then mix spinning back kicks into the sequence. Then, spinning hook kicks. Practice in super-slow motion. This aids your balance. After mixing all of your kicks at every height and angle, you are ready for dynamic wall stretches (Figures 1-39 to 1-41).
- Five Minutes of Wall Swings and Kicks: The purpose of using a wall is so you can brace yourself to kick higher than ever before. Hold onto a wall for balance.

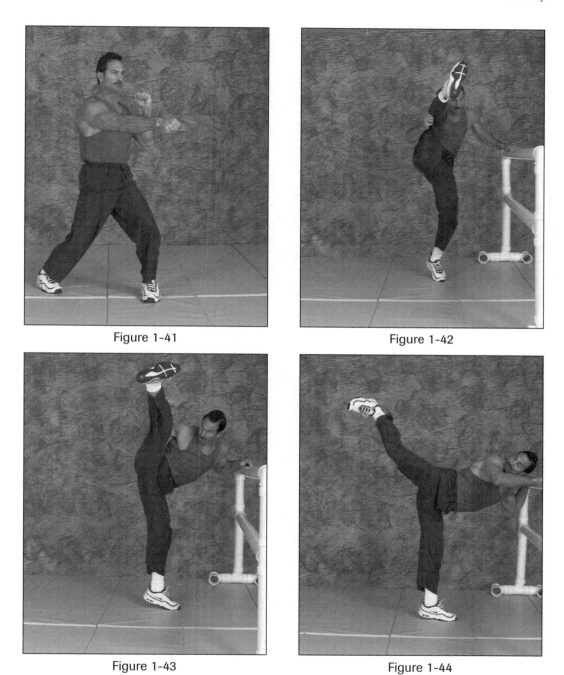

Figure 1-41

Figure 1-42

Figure 1-43

Figure 1-44

Step 1: Practice slow, controlled front, side, and back leg swings. Perform ten repetitions with each leg for each exercise (Figures 1-42 to1-44).

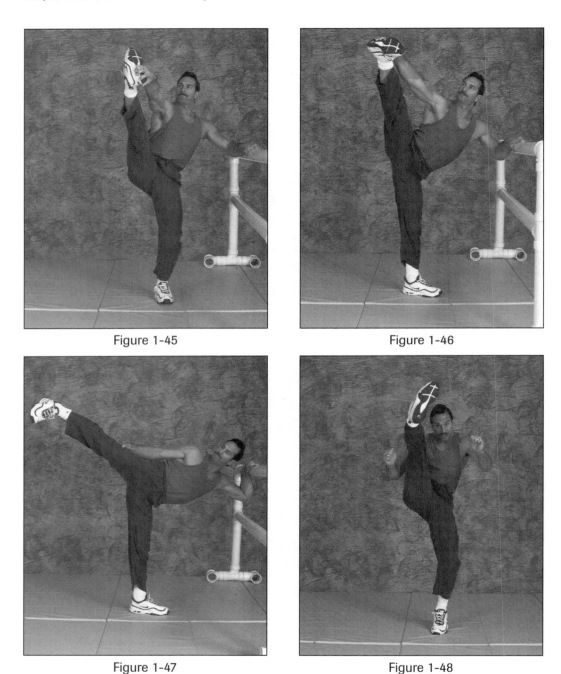

Figure 1-45

Figure 1-46

Figure 1-47

Figure 1-48

Step 2: Perform your leg swings, but instead of letting your leg drop, hold it with your free hand at maximum height for three seconds. Then let go (Figures 1-45 to 1-47).

Step 3: Use every ounce of your strength to keep your leg from dropping. Attempt to hold it with leg strength alone for three seconds, then relax (Figures 1-48 to 1-50).

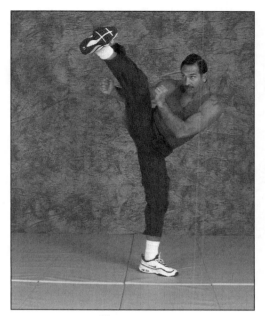

Figure 1-49

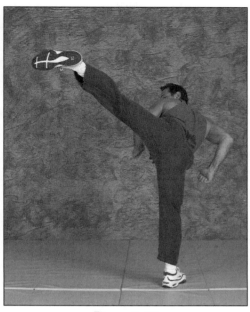

Figure 1-50

After your front, side, and back leg swings, you are ready to perform dynamic flexibility exercises for your roundhouse kick, side kick, and hook kick.

• Roundhouse Kick:

Step 1: Hold a wall for balance with your left hand and lift your right knee up to your side in a roundhouse kick fold position (Figure 1-51).

Step 2: Use your right hand to raise your knee a little higher. Let go with your hand and attempt to keep your knee up using the strength of your leg muscles (Figures 1-52 to 1-54).

Step 3: Without allowing your knee to drop perform ten consecutive roundhouse kicks. Switch sides and repeat with your left leg (Figure 1-55).

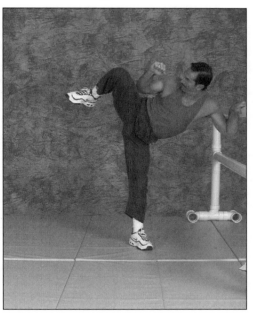

Figure 1-51

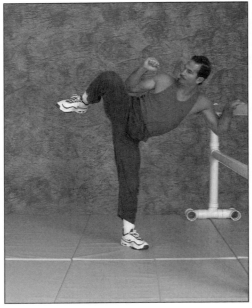

Figure 1-52

Figure 1-53

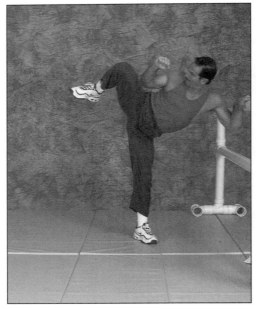

Figure 1-54

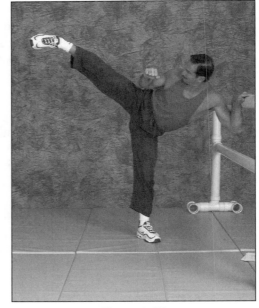

Figure 1-55

• Side Kick:

Step 1: Hold onto the wall with your left hand and lift your right knee into a side kick fold position (Figure 1-56).

Step 2: Use your right hand to add a little more inches of height. (Figures 1-57 and 1-58).

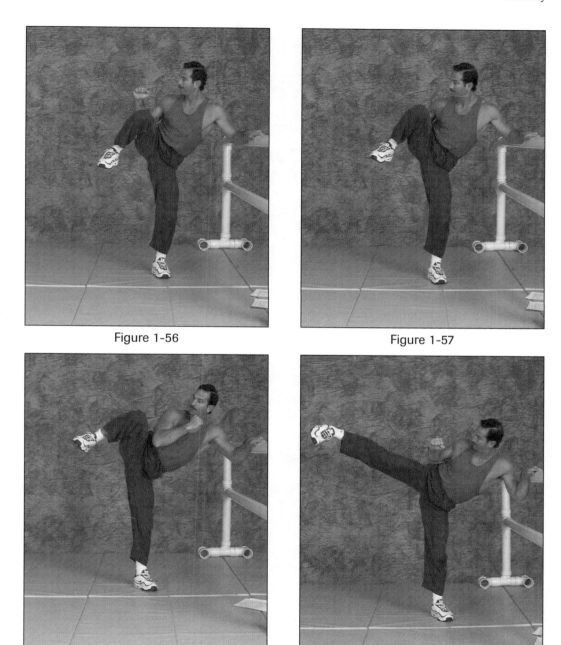

Figure 1-56

Figure 1-57

Figure 1-58

Figure 1-59

Step 3: Then throw ten consecutive side kicks without allowing your knee to drop. Switch sides and repeat with your left leg (Figure 1-59).

- Hook Kick:

  Step 1: Hold onto the wall with your left hand and lift your right knee into a hook kick fold position (Figure 1-60).

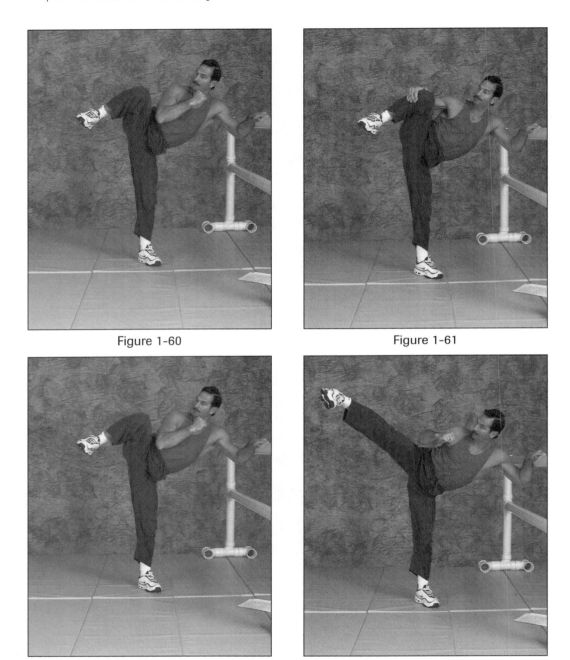

Figure 1-60

Figure 1-61

Figure 1-62

Figure 1-63

Step 2: Use your right hand to add a few more inches of height (Figures 1-61 and 1-62).

Step 3: Then throw ten consecutive side hook kicks without allowing your knee to drop. Switch sides and repeat with your left leg (Figure 1-63).

The purpose of these dynamic stretching exercises is to strengthen the opposing muscle groups at the end ranges of motion. Imagine how much easier it will be to throw perfect kicks if your muscles are strong enough to hold your leg in position until you complete your kick. No longer must you rely on momentum to blast a kick to its target. You can change the trajectory of your kicks at will, because now you will have the strength to do so. When an opening presents itself, you will find it. You can stretch your achilles tendon with a device such as that shown in Figure 1-64.

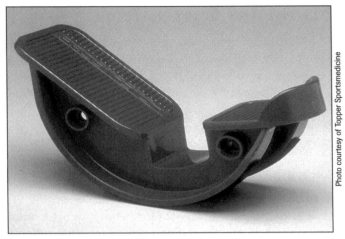

Figure 1-64

Photo courtesy of Topper Sportsmedicine

Substrate Usage

Each martial art has different requirements. Some demand speed and quickness. Others require impulsive movements with starts and stops, in a variety of directions.

But most martial arts, no matter what speed the performance requires, need a strong aerobic base. If a martial arts activity lasts from one to ten seconds such as a board break, or jab-punch-roundhouse kick combination, the enthusiast must rely on his adensosine triphosphate, phosphocreatine (ATP-PC) cycle for energy. This is a quick energy system used for high intensity activity. If the muscle cells were not previously "loaded" they will not perform maximally.

Any thirty to ninety second activity uses energy from your lactic acid system. Kata and sparring require thirty to ninety seconds of explosive action, followed by periods of rest. Remember how your legs felt when you were holding your back stance for ninety seconds? Soon the "burn" turned your legs into lead. Train your body to tolerate lactic acid by performing anaerobic, interval exercises such as plyometrics.

Martial arts activities longer than ninety seconds become aerobic. Find your "steady state." Steady state is that comfortable feeling you achieve after you warm up. Your body becomes accustomed to your workout. With every breath, you are supplying energy to your muscles. And because oxygen is your energy source, you can endure for long periods. You can improve your endurance in an aerobic kickboxing class.

Different martial artists have unique needs. Some folks want to tone muscle, others desire to lose fat. And a few hope to improve their martial arts skill. All of these needs may be addressed. The key is to keep your training programs simple, packed with a variety of aerobic and anaerobic activities, and most of all, fun.

Martial Arts Cross-Training

Martial arts cross-training is becoming increasingly popular. My martial arts cross-training program is designed to improve your martial arts performance.

Begin with a shadowboxing warm-up, followed by light stretching. Next perform a five minute abdominal routine, targeting your rectus abdominis, obliques, and transverse abdominis.

This serves as a warm up for weight training. Each day train a different muscle group. On Mondays work your back and biceps. Tuesdays, your chest and triceps. Wednesdays, your legs and shoulders. Never train a muscle group more than twice a week.

Following your weight training, perform a cardio-kickboxing bench aerobics routine. Vary the program daily.

At this point, your legs are sufficiently warmed, and you're ready for power plyometrics. Plyometrics consist of ten different jumping drills which enhance power. Then, jog and shuffle around the room, followed by combinations, kata, and sparring. Finish with heavy stretching and a cool-down.

Martial Arts Cardio Training—Strengthen Your Heart. Aerobic capacity is your body's ability to deliver oxygen to your working muscles. As you mature, your aerobic capacity decreases, but not as much if you continue to train in the martial arts. VO_2 max. is your muscle's ability to efficiently use nutrients from oxygen. World class martial artists are genetically gifted with a high VO_2 max.

If you train at the upper limits of your aerobic capacity you will perform favorably. Increase the pace of your martial arts training, but not too fast. Prevent deadening lactate from permeating your muscles. Lactic acid is that searing sensation as you exceed your anaerobic threshold. You reach your anaerobic threshold when your legs burn and you can hardly catch your breath. If you remain aerobic, but very close to your lactic acid/anaerobic threshold, you will kick harder and longer

Your aerobic capacity is not an issue if your goal is to complete a two hour martial arts class and lose fat. More important is the percent of your VO_2 max. you can maintain over a long period. This depends on your ability to tolerate lactate. A couple of days a week of quality martial arts interval training workouts may be your prescription for peak martial arts performance.

Sometimes you must "go anaerobic." Whether performing katas back to back, or sparring opponents in succession, you will feel lactate. This requires a physiological adjustment.

Martial Arts Heart Rate Training. When beginning to organize your martial arts workouts, it is important that you understand how your body's signals adapt and relate to the training drills that you are performing. Before we get into specifics let's discuss some basic terminology.

Heart Rates. Once you determine your resting heart rate and training heart rate, it will be easy to discover if you are working out too hard or too easy. After a few months of training, you will be amazed that you will probably be able to estimate your heart rate within a couple of beats.

For example during your warm up, your heart rate will may be around one hundred beats per minute. But when you accelerate into fast kicks, you will perceive that you are exerting more. Your training heart rate will correlate quite closely with how you feel.

Resting Heart Rate. This is your body's heart rate at rest, or your pulse rate taken approximately one hour before your normal waking time. This figure is one way to notice changes in your fitness and health levels.

Resting heart rate is very much genetic. Pro tennis player, Björn Borg had a resting heart rate of thirty-five beats per minute. Borg was in fabulous shape. But Olympic track star Jim Ryan, also in great shape, had a resting heart rate of seventy beats per minute.

Three ways to determine resting heart rate are:
- Have someone gently wake you up and then take your pulse one-hour before your normal waking hour. Count the pulse for one whole minute.
- In the evening, lie down in a supine position with some calming music and just allow your body to relax without any distractions and breathe comfortably for about twenty to thirty minutes. Count the pulse for one whole minute.
- Wear a heart rate monitor to sleep and glance at it just as you are starting to wake.

Record this number seven days in a row. Add them together, and divide by seven. This will give you a true average of your resting heart rate (RHR).

If you regularly record this figure and notice that your numbers are increasing by 10%, it means you are overtraining, overstressed, or your body is starting to break down and you could be starting to get ill. If you notice this happening, take the day off and pamper yourself by resting, getting a massage, or just train very light and easy for a couple of days until your RHR gets back to your normal average.

On the flip side, if you notice your RHR dropping slightly, that is one indication that your cardiovascular fitness level is improving. When this happens your heart has to beat less times within each minute to sustain your normal body functions.

Maximum Heart Rate. This is the maximum recommended number of times your heart can contract at any given minute. There are three ways to determine this:

- An easy, relatively accurate way to determine your maximum heart rate (MHR) is by using this age-predicted formula: 220–age=MHR (for men), 226–age=MHR (for women).
- This next method is found in *The Heart Rate Monitor Book* by Sally Edwards. She suggests performing a series of sprints after warming up. Give all-out, extreme effort until your heart rate reading no longer rises and you approach exhaustion. The final number is your maximum heart rate. Obviously a heart rate monitor must be used and supervision by a medical professional should be observed. This method is definitely not recommended for beginner martial artists or sedentary individuals.
- A maximum stress test performed by a physician in a clinical setting is your third approach. A maximum stress test requires you to walk on a treadmill while a doctor measures all of your vital signs. The walk turns into a jog, and into a run however, as the treadmill speeds up, and so does the grade. Soon you can barely breathe as you are moving your feet as quickly as you can. Your doctor keeps asking, "Are you

okay?" and you are supposed to nod Yes as you push yourself to your limit. At the moment you reached your limit, you achieved your maximum heart rate.

Recovery Heart Rate. This is the heart rate typically determined two minutes after the your martial arts workout is finished. Determine your recovery heart rate (RHR) by counting your pulse for one minute.

The only difference between recovery heart rate and resting heart rate is that your recovery measure is taken after exercise. Record this number frequently since it is another method of determining cardiovascular fitness. The quicker the number drops the better your condition.

Training Zones. There are two training zones that we will be concerned with in your martial arts. The start up or recovery training zone and the improved fitness or higher caloric expenditure zone. When you know your training zones, you can increase or decrease your martial arts workload accordingly.

For example, if your recovery-training zone is 80 to 100 beats per minute, and your actual heart rate is 120, you should decrease your intensity. And if your improved fitness zone is 140 to 170 beats per minute, and your heart rate monitor shows that you are working out at 190 beats per minute, once again you should slow down.

1. The start-up or recovery training zone is 50%–70% of MHR. Determine zone by using this formula:
   _____(MHR) x 0.50 = _____Low end figure
   _____(MHR) x 0.70 = _____High end figure
   Example for a forty year old martial artist with a MHR of 180
   180 x 0.50 = 90
   180 x 0.70 = 126

So, this martial artist's start-up or recovery training zone is 90–126 beats per minute. She should allow her heart rate to drop to this level during the warm up, between kicking intervals, and during the cool down. If her heart rate is higher than 126 beats per minute, she should slow down.

2. The working zone or higher caloric expenditure zone is 70%–90% of MHR. Determine zone by using this formula:
   _____(MHR) x 0.70 = _____Low end figure
   _____(MHR) x 0.90 = _____High end figure
   Example for a forty year old martial artist with a MHR of 180
   180 x 0.70 = 126
   180 x 0.90 = 162

So, this martial artist's working zone or higher caloric expenditure zone is 126-162 beats per minute.

Intervals. Interval training is varying your intensity throughout your martial arts session. Alternate high-intensity work bouts and low-intensity rest periods. Intervals are used to improve your martial arts performance using effort intervals followed by recovery intervals.

You can make interval training specific to your martial arts goals by practicing a specific punch or kick. Or you can use intervals to improve your fitness. To begin, make intervals equal to your normal steady state program. Follow this with a rest/recovery segment performed at a lower intensity.

Research has shown that interval training improves both your aerobic and anaerobic capacity. Continuous, long, slow, martial arts training improves aerobic capacity only.

Martial arts interval training has also been shown to burn more total fat and calories than continuous training. Intervals allow you to perform more work increasing your Exercise Post Oxygen Consumption (EPOC). EPOC, the "afterburn", is the absolute number of calories you consume, long after you have completed your martial arts workout.

Intervals have the potential to train your heart muscle longer and more effectively than a single bout of continuous martial arts training. During interval training, your heart must overcome a greater resistance. This leads to improved venous return, which results in greater ventricular filling and contractility. You experience a more complete emptying which increases your stroke volume and cardiac output.

Interval training also improves your muscle's ability to tolerate lactic acid. You become accustomed to short periods of kicking and punching just below your anaerobic threshold. This helps you learn to delay the onset of fatigue during sparring and kata.

If you have a heart rate monitor, use the information presented in the heart rate section to correlate your heart rate to your perceived exertion.

Beginning Martial Arts Interval Training. A martial arts aerobic interval-training program is low intensity but continues for longer than three minutes. Both the work and rest intervals occur at an intensity that is within your aerobic system. The interval period is performed at a slightly higher intensity than your steady state. The rest period is slightly lower than your steady state. The time in each interval usually ranges anywhere from four to fifteen minutes.

Intermediate Martial Arts Interval Training. Put on your dobok. Spend five minutes shadow boxing at an easy pace. Then gradually increase your intensity until you are punching and kicking at about seventy percent of your maximum speed. You may feel a slight burn in your legs. And your lungs may open up for the first time in years. Hold this pace for about a minute. Then slow down to your normal tempo for two minutes. Increase your speed again to seventy percent for another leg exploding, lung expanding, minute. Cool down to a relaxed pace for another five.

Use intervals for kicking, punching, or blocking techniques. The faster, more intense, pace may be uncomfortable at first. Your heart rate and breathing will skyrocket. Soon you will crave it. Add one one-minute interval each week until you are punching, kicking, or blocking a maximum of ten one-minute cycles. If you do not relish watching the clock, simply speed up when you feel like it. Then slow to your normal rate until you are energized again. Interval training burns fat, builds endurance, speed, and recovery. You will complete your workout sooner, and it is a pleasant change of pace.

Advanced Martial Arts Intervals. An advanced interval training program (ATP-PC) is very high intensity, and short in duration (one to fifteen seconds). Kick or punch a heavy bag at ninety-five percent intensity for fifteen seconds. Then take a forty-five second break. Your recovery interval is absolute-rest to allow for replacement of ATP and creatine phosphate. Because your work/rest cycle is relatively short, you can repeat the cycle ten to twenty times within a single workout.

Another advanced interval training program (lactic acid system) kicks in at a high intensity and short duration (forty-five to ninety seconds). The work interval is greater than your anaerobic threshold. After your warm up, do a kata at sixty-five percent of your maximum speed. Then recover by doing slow footwork drills. Your rest interval occurs in the aerobic system. Use this program if you are highly fit and athletic. Your rest interval is active recovery. This allows for removal of lactic acid.

Speedplay is a form of interval training that is based on how you feel. It is less systematized than normal intervals. You govern how hard you want to work. You control your intensity based on your tolerance. Speedplay may be more enjoyable than timed intervals. It teaches beginning martial artists how to progress beyond their anaerobic threshold. They learn to subjectively rate their perceived exertion.

Circuit Martial Arts Intervals. Martial arts intervals may be performed on a circuit. Perform one set of twenty repetitions of kicks at sixty percent of your maximum. Take about thirty seconds to finish. Your rest interval is the period between exercises. Recovery time is minimal, as it includes only the seconds required to regain your energy for your next technique. Your goal is to complete twenty repetitions on all kicks machines with limited rest between sets.

A variation of circuit kick training is aerobic circuit training. Aerobic circuit training is simply adding a thirty-second to three-minute aerobics workout between each kicking set. For example, you might do thirty seconds to three minutes of jumping jacks between each set of kicks.

Studies demonstrate metabolism remains elevated up to fifteen hours after a martial arts interval training session. One investigation examined a group who trained moderately four times a week burning four hundred calories per session. Another group trained moderately twice a week, but on the other two days performed interval training. The intervals only burned 250 calories per session, but two days of moderate exercise combined with two days of intervals incinerated nine times more fat than four days of moderate exercise.

Martial Arts Intervals—Safety & Speed. The benefits of interval training include:

1. Increasing your VO_2 maximum. You will also be able to work out at a higher percentage of your VO_2 max. because you will increase your anaerobic threshold.
2. You can burn more total fat and calories in a shorter workout session thereby maximizing the use of your time.
3. You will be effectively stimulating both fast and slow twitch muscle fibers.
4. You can change your interval routine to avoid overuse injuries.
5. Intervals spice up your program.

CHAPTER TWO

Understanding Your Body

Your Back

To examine your flexibility and balance, lie flat on a hard floor (Figure 2-1). Where do you feel the heaviest pressure against the floor?

Stand barefoot facing a mirror (Figure 2-2). How is your weight distributed? Are your feet angled? Are your hips even? Are your shoulders level and parallel with your hips? Do your toes and kneecaps face forward? Do you see the sides or back of your hands?

Bend your index finger back until it feels uncomfortable. An X-ray won't show what is causing your pain. When you return your finger back to normal, it feels fine. Similarly, some postures make your back "unhappy."

When a random sampling of subjects were required to have their backs X-rayed, some showed abnormalities and others did not. Amazingly, some of the folks with and spondy-

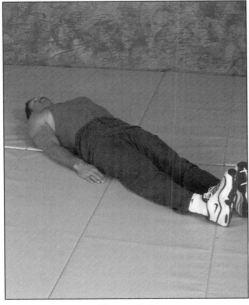

Figure 2-1

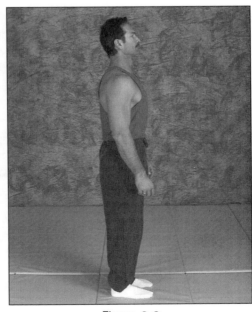

Figure 2-2

lolisthesis were pain free. Others, who complained of severe back pain, showed no sign of deformity.

Weak abdominals are not always to blame for low back pain. Usually tight hamstrings are the culprit. Fitness testing in a later chapter may help determine the origin of your pain. If you score high in the bent knee curl-up test, but low on the sit and reach trunk flexion test, focus on improving your hamstring flexibility. Muscles can be short or overtight from disuse.

Poor fitness leads to poor posture. If you carry most of your weight in your abdomen, your back muscles must counterbalance. The same is true concerning the relationship between your quadriceps and hamstrings. Your hamstrings should be at least sixty percent as strong as your quadriceps (thigh muscles). Tight hip flexors and hamstrings, combined with weak abdominals and upper back may be a prime cause for your suffering.

Drop this book on the floor. Bend down to pick it up. You probably twisted in your chair and leaned over sideways from your waist. Unsupported forward flexion with a shearing diagonal force is unhealthy for the disks in your low back.

Your disks are collagen packets filled with water. You are taller in the morning because your disks are not compressed from hours of daily standing or sitting. When you wake up, sit on the potty, and proceed directly into your abdominal training, your inflated disks may protrude into your spinal nerve causing pain. Therefore, perform your crunches later in the day.

Does your back hurt when you walk? Walking loads and unloads your disks, like a massage. With most muscular problems, moving around helps to relieve pain. But more serious ailments could be aggravated while walking or moving. This may be due to a nerve impingement or herniated disk. In these cases, walking exacerbates pain because of nerve involvement. Pulsing and throbbing pain, or temperature disturbances may be a vascular issue.

Bend forward from your waist. At about fifteen degrees of flexion your back muscles (erector spinae, quadratus laborum) eccentrically lengthen. When you bend to about forty-five degrees your hips take over. Bend past ninety degrees and your back is supported by ligaments (Figures 2-3 to 2-5). Pain receptors called nociceptors are in these ligaments.

Sit in your chair with your left leg on the floor and your right ankle crossed over your left knee in a figure-4 position. Slowly bring your chest toward your right knee. Did you feel pain? Try your other leg (Figures 2-6 to 2-7). Disc injuries, muscular imbalances, lack of flexibility in the gluteals and piriformis (muscle under your hip) can create sciatic nerve problems. Check with your doctor if you feel tingling or numbness radiating down your leg.

Other stretches may relieve your low back pain:
1. Lie on your back and bring your knees to your chest in a fetal position (Figure 2-8). This stretches your erector spinae and quadratus laborum.
2. Lift one knee to your chest and grab it with your arms. Let your other leg remain on the floor. Switch legs and repeat (Figure 2-9). This stretches your hip flexor muscles.

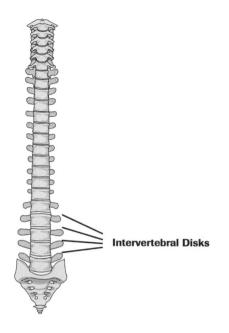

Intervertebral Disks

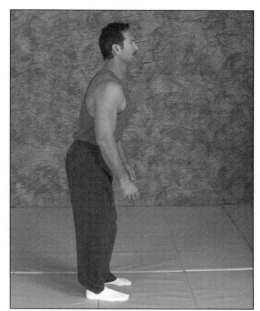

Figure 2-3

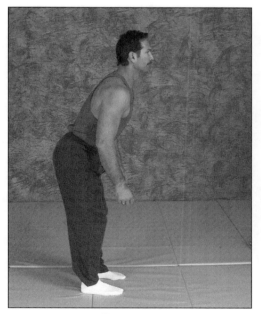

Figure 2-4

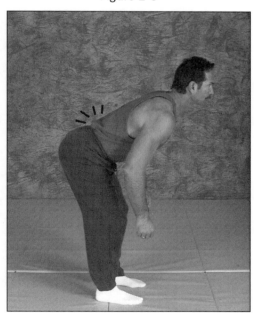

Figure 2-5

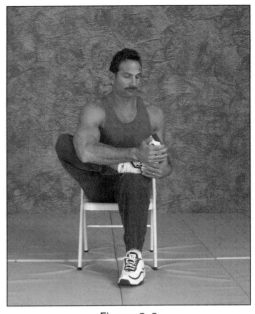

Figure 2-6

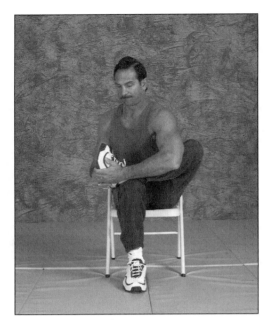

Figure 2-7

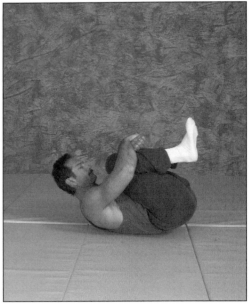

Figure 2-8

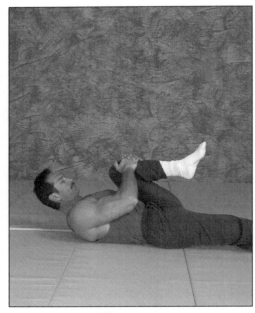

Figure 2-9

3. Lean sideways into a wall keeping your pelvis stable. Bend sideways not forward (Figure 2-10). This may help if you have a disk that protrudes sideways.

4. Sit in your chair and slowly twist sideways maintaining a neutral spine throughout (Figures 2-11 and 2-12). This may relieve pressure on your disks.

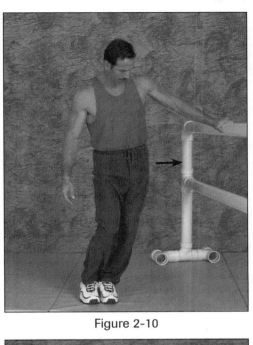

Figure 2-10

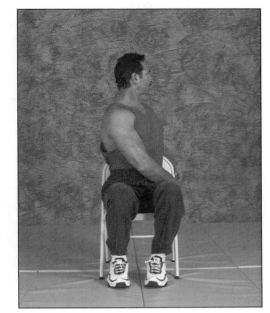

Figure 2-11

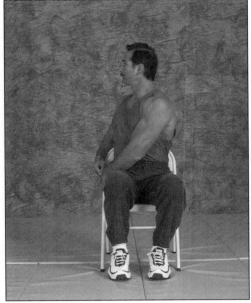

Figure 2-12

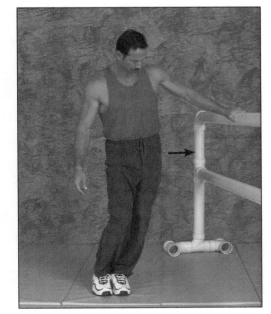

Figure 2-13

5. Lie on your stomach. Raise your right arm and your left leg. Raise your left arm and right leg (Figures 2-13 to 2-15). This "Superman" exercise strengthens your erector spinae and quadratus laborum in your back.

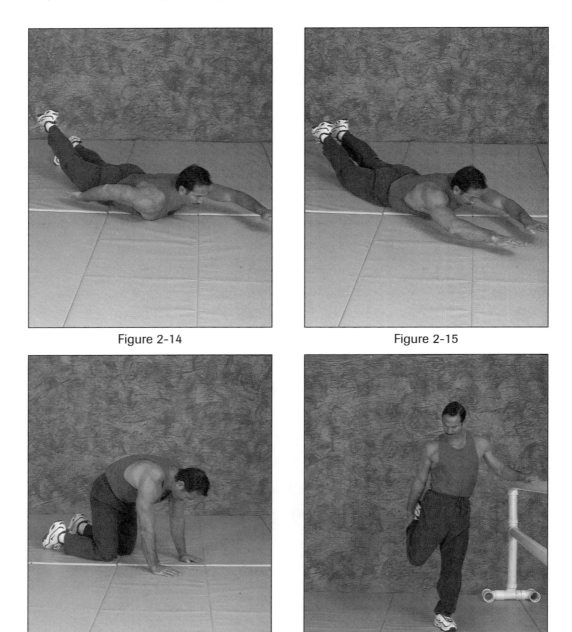

Figure 2-14

Figure 2-15

Figure 2-16

Figure 2-17

6. Roll over onto your hands and knees (Figure 2-16). Lift your upper back and stretch resembling a "mad cat". Hold this stretch for three seconds.

7. Stand with your right hand against a wall. Grab the top of your left foot with your left hand. Bend your left knee until you feel a stretch in your left quadriceps. Switch legs and repeat (Figure 2-17).

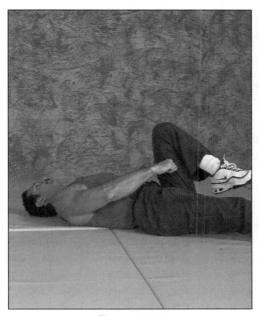

Figure 2-18

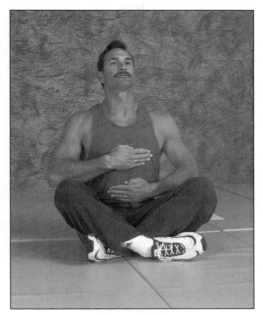

Figure 2-19

Strength. It is not beneficial to possess awesome abs at the expense of awesome low back pain. I have seen people do bizarre exercises in the gym in an attempt to gain awesome abs. One young man placed a twenty five-pound weight on his face while he performed sit-ups. His nose protruded through the hole in the middle of the plate so he could breathe.

If your lower back hurts, begin with trunk stabilization movements. Lie on your back and lift your arm and opposite knee toward your chest while maintaining a neutral spine. Next perform pelvic tilts. To perform a pelvic tilt, place your palms over your abdomen and chest so that the pinky of one hand is above the thumb of the other (Figures 2-18 to 2-20). Those fingers do not touch each other while you are in a relaxed position. When you posteriorly tilt your pelvis your pinky and thumb touch.

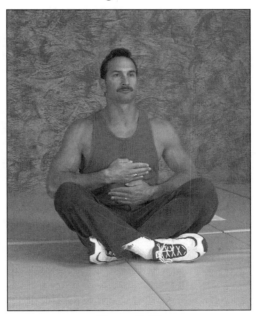

Figure 2-20

Performing hundreds of crunches a day may be harmful to your disks. Crunching forward forces the annulus of lower back disks into your spinal nerve causing pain. After you finish your abdominal workout, perform some hyperextensions to move your lower back disk material back into place.

Your abdominal wall is thinner toward your ribs near your solar plexus. That is one reason the upper part of your rectus abdominus fatigues quickly when you perform crunches. Your hip flexors do most of the work when you execute reverse crunches. It feels as if you are training your lower abdomen, but it is simply the close proximity of your hip flexors to your rectus abdominus. Consider it a case of referred soreness.

Test the balance of strength between your lower back and abdominal muscles by performing the following exercise. Lie on your back and keep your lower back flat while you extend your legs toward the ceiling. Slowly drop your legs while attempting to hold your lower back flat to the floor. If you can pull this off, your abdominals are strong enough to counter the pull from your hip flexors.

When you develop powerful obliques (the abdominal muscles on the sides of your torso), you receive an added bonus of muscular love handles over your hips. Training obliques does not make your waist smaller. In fact if you overload your muscles, your waist may grow larger.

When your abdominals contract they produce an inner tube like effect to stabilize your torso. When you contract your obliques you provide structural support to your spine as if filling an inner tube.

In aerobics classes, instructors discipled you to "pull your belly button to your spine" to protect your lower back. Ironically it is not your abdominals that hold your belly button in, it is your diaphragm. A preferred guideline is to maintain a neutral spine when performing your abdominals. A neutral spine is a slight arch in your low back. If you own a large buttocks you may be incapable of holding your lower back to the floor. If you have a heavy chest or thick legs, crunches and reverse crunches are difficult.

Back Pain. Low back pain may be caused by weakness in your abdominals or lower back muscles. It may be tightness in your hamstrings or hip flexors. Or you might have a structural problem such as scoliosis (S-curve), no curve, or bone degeneration. Screenings such as trunk flexibility tests, hamstring flexibility tests, and bent knee curl up tests can help to determine the problem. A leg length discrepancy may cause pain on one side of your back. Good posture while sitting and bad posture while standing could be an indication for leg length problems.

- Osteoarthritis: bone degeneration may cause nerve impingement. Perform pelvic tilts from a chair or against a wall.

- Rheumatoid arthritis: shows up in bone deformities in your legs and hips, which may affect your lower back. Do not exercise if you are in pain. Adjust your range of motion so it does not elevate pain in your deformed joint.

- Fibromyalgia: feels as if you have the aches and pains of flu without the fever. It has been described as arthritis of the muscles. Good form and moderation is important in your abdominal program if you suffer from fibromyalgia.

- Osteoporosis: modify your abdominal exercise to eliminate the hunching forward of your shoulders; the position your are degenerating towards. Pelvic tilts in a chair, against a wall, or on the floor, are indicated if your osteoporosis is severe. If it has not progressed, regular exercises are fine but incorporate chest stretches.

Preventing and Handling Low Back Pain. Back pain is treated differently now than ten years ago. Grandparents hurt their backs and went to bed. Doctors prescribed bed rest and narcotic pain killers. This lead to strength, endurance, and muscle loss.

Recent research demonstrated that prolonged bed rest has no benefit, and actually hinders recovery. Specifically, a study showed that 186 patients given two days of bed rest recovered slower than a control group who were told to continue their normal day-to-day activities.

Today, treatment for back pain is active recovery. The goal is to improve function quickly, before muscles atrophy and tighten.

Nonsteroidal anti-inflammatories are recommended for acute pain and inflammation. But these drugs should not be continued longer than twelve weeks because of possible harmful side effects.

The disks in your spine are collagen packets filled with fluid. They are fed by solute transported during your normal activities. Simply moving around pumps liquid through your disks. It keeps them hydrated. If you lie flat on your back for extended lengths of time, you jeopardize nourishment to your disks. That is why immobility increases back pain.

A vicious cycle occurs when your back hurts. You lie down in bed. Your muscles atrophy. Your connective tissues and muscles shorten. Your aerobic fitness deteriorates. When your aerobic level decreases your pain levels increase. A study of 1,652 firefighters in Los Angeles revealed that back injuries were ten times higher among those who were least aerobically fit.

> ## Low Back Martial Arts Training Tips:
>
> 1. Move from one stance to the next comfortably with a slight arch in your lower back. Keep your abdominal muscles firm and breathe from your diaphragm.
>
> 2. Warm up before you perform any vigorous martial arts exercise.
>
> 3. You may feel slight discomfort as you train. If you feel a sharp pain in your lower back, you are pushing too hard.

There are other reasons martial arts training may prevent low back pain. Martial arts training helps to decrease fat around your middle. Less fat on your tummy places less stress on your lumbar spine.

And while you are doing martial arts, you are increasing your endorphins. Endorphins are pain-relieving chemicals released in your brain when you train. These chemicals provide a "natural high" which alters your perception of pain and helps decrease anxiety and depression.

Tai Chi loads and unloads your disks in a gentle massage to aid healing. Slow rhythmic martial arts type movements strengthen your lumbar flexors and extensors in a natural, balanced way. These exercises do not require repeated pounding or shearing forces caused by anaerobic activities such as racquetball and heavy weight lifting.

There has not been enough research to determine which type of martial arts are best for preventing low back pain. One study showed that sedentary women were motivated to perform intensive, dynamic, vigorous exercises like fast kata. Blue-collar males reduced pain by doing isometric exercises such as stance training for their legs and trunk.

Stretching and strengthening muscles in your trunk reduces the chances of having another acute attack of back pain. Your main goal of martial arts training is to balance the strength between your abdominal muscles and your back muscles. If your back hurts when you perform crunches or hyperextensions, simply perform isometrics.

Isometrics allow you to contract muscles without moving them. Sit back so your lower back is flat against your chair. Notice that as you flattened your back, your abdominals isometrically contracted (Figure 2-21).

You can do the same for your back muscles by lying on your stomach. Raise your right arm out to the front and your left leg to the back. Switch arms and legs. Then raise both arms and both legs simultaneously. If these exercises are painful, limit the range of motion so you are barely moving. Just contract the muscles.

Crunch type exercises are contraindicated for people with bulging disks. Each time you

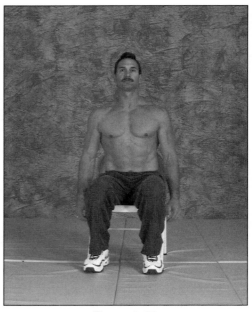

Figure 2-21

flex your spine you may be pressing your disk against the spinal nerve, increasing pain. Therefore, if you are diagnosed with a disk problem, concentrate on extension movements.

After several months of stretching and strengthening, there should be some remission of pain. If not, mind/body stress management techniques may be an option.

Clinical depression and high levels of anxiety may contribute to low back pain. Surgery is a last resort and is suggested only after conservative measures have been used. Statistically, only one percent of back pain cases require surgery.

Abdominal Support. The location and design of your abdominal muscles affect their function. Lying on your back doing sit-ups strengthens your hip flexors and rectus abdominis (a.k.a. six pack).

But sit-ups do little to equalize the strength in your obliques and back. Humans stand in an upright posture. Your abdominal muscles stabilize your movement.

Stand and place your hands around your waist. Move in any direction. You do not have to move far before you feel your abdominals brace your effort.

Train your abdominals with crunches. And practice contracting them during your normal, upright posture. Why? Because most of your daily activities are performed while standing or seated. Electromyography studies demonstrated that your obliques (side of your stomach muscles) are active when you are standing.

Improve the balance and strength in your trunk. Build your back and abdominal muscles from the inside out. Rather than just worrying about a "six pack," train your core for internal stability.

The safest position for your lower back is a neutral spine. Neutral simply means a slight curve in your lower back. A neutral spine places the least amount of pressure on your disks,

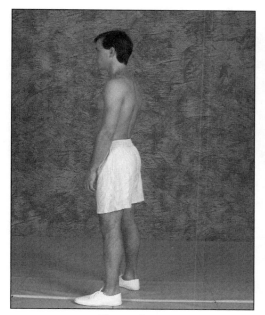

Figure 2-22

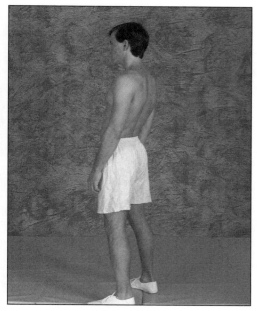

Figure 2-23

ligaments, and bones. You can absorb impact better. The breadth of your lordotic curve is individual, like a fingerprint (Figure 2-22).

Excessive arching and flattening of your back stresses your spinal disks. This can lead to nerve root irritation, degeneration of the vertebrae, and herniated discs. Chronic pain may be caused by gravity pulling you out of alignment while you are sitting or standing (Figures 2-23 and 2-24).

Develop a strong midsection, but not at the expense of a painful back. Crunches performed with a flat back are effective, but return to neutral after each repetition to maintain functional stability.

Do your crunches, and pay attention to your spine. Contract your stabilizers to stay in neutral. Although neutral is best, it is difficult to maintain.

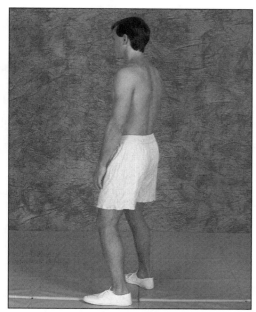

Figure 2-24

In minutes, gravity and a variety of other factors pull you out of your perfect alignment. It takes practice and muscular endurance to stay in neutral. Try spending five minutes in neutral. Add two minutes a week until you can sit through your favorite sitcom in neutral.

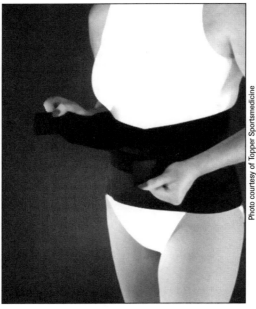

Photo courtesy of Topper Sportsmedicine

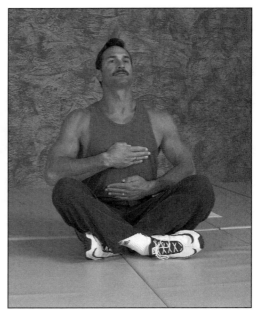

| Figure 2-25 | Figure 2-26 |

Practice your neutral spine while sitting, standing, and exercising. While reading, think "posture." Adjust your spine into pelvic neutrality. Notice how healthy it feels to release unwanted tension.

Your torso is the connection between your upper and lower limbs when you perform any martial arts technique. A synergy between body parts provide stability. A powerful core allows you to train your entire physique with less likelihood of injury. Acute back injuries occur from failing to stabilize your torso when you are trying to move heavy objects. Belts may help you become aware of your posture during lifting (Figure 2-25).

Traditional abdominal fitness evaluations concentrate on sit ups or crunches. Excellent scores are given to individuals who bounce through hundreds of repetitions. Sit-ups actually test power and speed.

A more useful measure of a strong torso might be one that demonstrates abdominal stability. Lie on your back. Bring your feet together with your knees straight. Point your legs up to a ninety degree position. Slowly attempt to drop your legs, holding your lower back flat to the floor.

Your hip flexors eccentrically contract against your

Do's and Don'ts for abdominal exercise:

- Do contract your abdominal muscles.
- Don't hold your breath.
- Don't arch your back too much, keep a neutral spine.
- Don't pull on your neck.
- Do use slow and controlled movements.
- Don't swing your legs.
- Don't continue repetitions if you lose your form.

abdominals. And your back must resist the downward force of your legs. As soon as your back begins to arch, mark your score.

If your legs only moved a few inches (seventy degree angle), you displayed poor abdominal stability (Figures 2-26 to 2-28). If your legs reached almost all the way to the floor (five degree angle), your torso strength was excellent.

You may be capable of completing one hundred sit-ups in a couple of minutes. But without abdominal strength, stability, and balance, you may not be able to move your legs more than a few inches without your low back curling off the floor.

Your external and internal obliques are movers and stabilizers of your torso. When you twist for a reverse punch, or lean sideways to evade an attack, your obliques control your motion. Lateral curls, which work the lateral fibers of your obliques, should be part of your training.

Your goal is not absolute abdominal strength. You probably do not plan to enter a sit up contest bearing a one hundred pound weight on your chest. And when was the last time you tossed a fifty pound Frisbee?

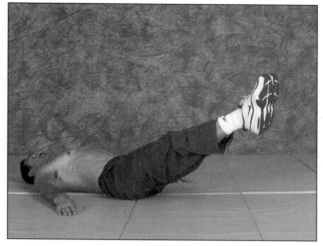

Figure 2-27

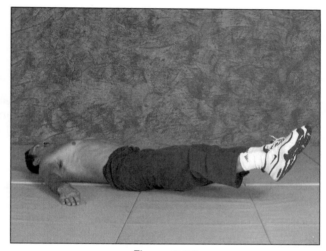

Figure 2-28

You must rely on torso endurance to spar for twenty minutes, however. Twisting in your chair to answer a phone, or reaching to retrieve a paperclip activates your internal and external obliques.

Your Elbow

Tennis elbow can affect you even though you are a martial artist and not a tennis player. This injury, termed lateral epicondylitis, is an overuse injury of the tendon that attaches the forearm's extensor muscles to the elbow at its bony outer knob, the lateral epicondyle.

With repeated stress from punching, striking, and blocking, the tendon can suffer microtears that cause the elbow to become tender and inflamed.

If you have tennis elbow, avoid lifting objects with your hand in the palm down position. Also, try wearing a counterforce band around your upper forearm during your martial arts training. This allows shock to be absorbed in the band rather than farther up at the epicondyle.

Anti-inflammatories are recommended, and so is ice. Some patients receive steroid injections. Tennis elbow is slow in healing, sometimes taking from eight weeks to a year to become pain free.

Tennis elbow involves damage to your forearm muscles and tendons. Your first preventive measure is to keep your elbow "soft" at all times. That is, be sure not to lock your elbow on any punch, strike, or block. Ice your elbow for ten to twenty minutes after each martial arts training session.

Do not cause pain. If any strike, punch or block causes pain, modify it by changing the range of motion.

Listen to your body. Pain is your body's way of saying: "Rest me!" Rest means to use the elbow for all of your normal activities, unless there is pain.

Your Shoulders

Because your shoulder can move in seven quadrants, it has the greatest range of motion of any joint in your body. No other joint is as flexible, and unstable as the shoulder.

The shoulder (glenohumeral [GH]) joint is a shallow ball and socket variety that allows your arm to move freely in all directions to block and strike. Your shoulder, therefore, depends heavily on the surrounding muscles to provide necessary stability.

The shoulder joint consists of the ball of the humerus (upper arm) and the socket (glenoid) of the scapula (shoulder blade). The surrounding capsule allows a wide range of movement. The place where the humerus articulates with the glenoid is reinforced by a fibrocartilage collar, which increases the stability of the shoulder.

Four short rotator cuff muscles and their tendons surround the joint and contribute towards its stability. The rotator cuff muscles are small, but play an important role in shoulder stabilization. These four rotator cuff muscles include your supraspinatus, infraspinatus, teres minor, and subscapularis. Together they have an essential steadying effect on the head of the humerus.

A fluid filled bursae sac acts as a shock absorber for your shoulder joint. If it is inflamed it bulges and becomes, thick, scarred, and painful. This is your body's way of letting you know that you should discontinue the heavy bag work that created inflammation in the first place.

Pain also has an inhibiting effect on muscle. Your rotator cuff muscles waste away (atrophy) within a short time. Other muscles take over in an attempt to alleviate the pain.

Rotator cuff problems may be attributed to the soft ligamentous structures that attach the ball to the socket. Imagine a big ball balancing on the end of a seal's nose. Compare that to the ball and socket joint of your shoulder. If the ball moves around too much in the socket, it may ride to high (subluxate).

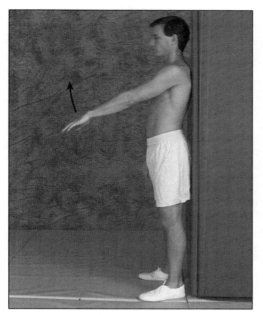

Figure 2-29

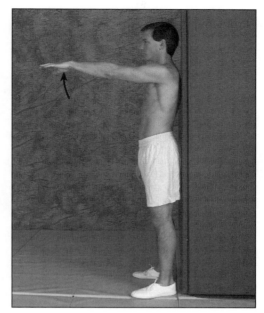

Figure 2-30

The worst case scenario is that it comes out of the socket and dislocates. At the pre-World Taekwondo Championships in Taiwan, I witnessed a Chinese fighter throw a punch and yell a blood-curdling scream. He had dislocated his shoulder. Without missing a beat, he used his other hand to place his limp, dislocated arm into his dobok as a sling.

Another analogy to help you understand the importance of your rotators is to visualize a tent. Your upper arm is a tent pole, extending from the ground. Your shoulder is the place on the ground where the pole sits. Your rotator cuff muscles are the ropes that secure the tent pole. If these ropes remain strong and in place, the pole maintains its proper position, and the tent does not collapse. However if any of the ropes stretch, loosen, or snap, the remaining ropes will tug the pole out of position and the tent will fail.

Your rotator cuff muscles hold your ball in your GH socket when you cock your arm to throw a knife hand strike, and when you follow through on your punches.

Martial artists train their pectoral muscles (chest) for cosmetic value, but many do not take the time to strengthen their invisible rotator cuff muscles. When you throw a punch, your shoulder joint funnels any motion from the ground and channels the force.

A martial artist uses his legs for power, and gets sixty percent of his power from his hips. Your shoulder may be the weak link in your power chain. Although it does not take enormous strength to throw a punch, conditioning and endurance are necessary.

Preventing and Handling Shoulder Problems. Stand with your scapula (shoulder blades) against a wall. Attempt to raise your affected arm to shoulder height, parallel to the floor (Figures 2-29 and 2-30). If you cannot do so without moving your scapula or trapezius (muscles on the top of your shoulder beside your neck), you may have a rotator cuff injury.

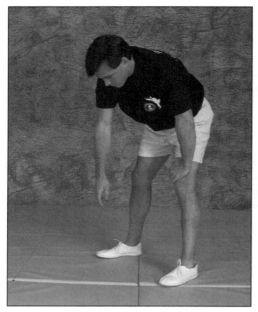

Figure 2-31

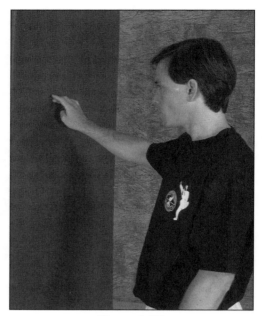

Figure 2-32

There is a poor supply of blood to your rotator cuff. That is one reason it is slow to heal. If you have a rotator cuff injury, your goal is to improve blood flow to that area by performing passive range of motion (ROM) exercises.

1. The first exercise your physical therapist may provide for you is the pendulum swing. Simply bend over and support yourself from the waist with your uninjured arm. Gently rotate your injured arm in a circular motion allowing momentum to create the movement (Figure 2-31).

2. The next exercise requires you to let your fingers do the walking. Walk up and down a wall using your fingertips. Press your fingertips against the wall for balance. Walk around the

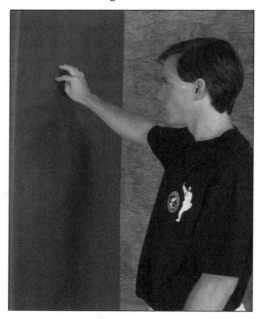

Figure 2-33

wall with your fingertips (Figures 2-32 and 2-33). This is an exercise to strengthen your rotator muscles while maintaining stability.

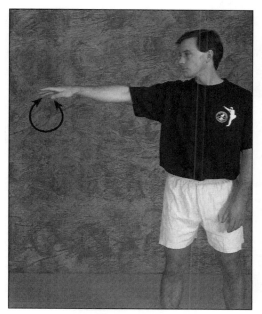

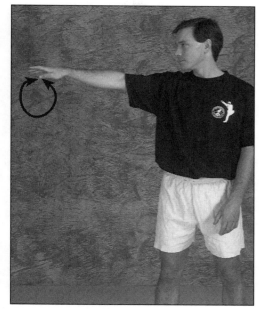

Figure 2-34   Figure 2-35

3. Finally you are ready for unweighted arm circles. Move your arms in a small ROM, gently strengthening your rotator muscles (Figures 2-34 and 2-35).

Push-ups—How to Perform Them Properly to Protect Your Shoulders. Your body is an incredible machine. Your muscles and bones become stronger the more you use them. And martial artists are notorious for their push-up routines. I watched sixty year old Jhoon Rhee perform one hundred push-ups in one hundred seconds.

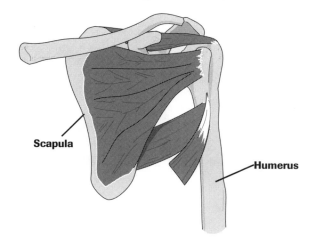

Perform mechanically correct push-ups to prevent a shoulder breakdown. A repetitive, biomechanically risky push-up might lead to joint degeneration over time. Or worse, an acute injury that would be devastating.

A proper push-up is performed from the floor, with your hands a little less than shoulder width apart. Hold your arms close to your body as you press up. Do not lock your elbows in the up position. Keep your back straight with a slight arch in your lower spine (Figures 2-36 and 2-37). Your neck supports your head in a neutral position.

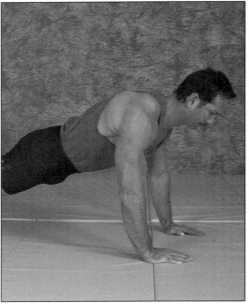

Figure 2-36

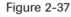

Figure 2-37

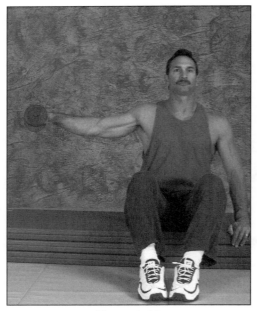

Figure 2-38

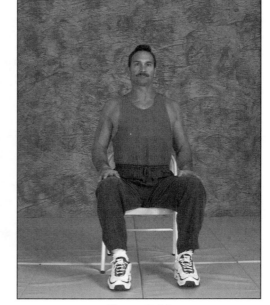

Figure 2-39

Push-ups train muscles in your shoulders, upper arms, and a collection of stabilizer muscles in your back and abdominals. In order to understand the mechanics of your shoulder anatomy during push-ups, let's review some physiology.

Your scapulae (shoulder blades) and glenohumeral (ball and socket) joint are involved. If you lift your arm out to the side as in shoulder abduction, your scapula rotates upward and so does your glenohumeral joint in a rhythmic, synergistic fashion (Figure 2-38).

Pull your shoulder blades together as in scapular retraction, which simulates the down phase of a push-up (Figure 2-39). Here you are adducting your scapula.

Push forward with your hands and move your scapulae apart. This is comparable to the up phase of a push-up, and is referred to as scapular protraction. This is also termed scapular abduction. Scapular adduction and abduction utilize different muscles than shoulder (glenohumeral) joint action.

Your scapulae have posterior (back of the body) and anterior (front of the body) muscles that control their movement.

Posterior muscles include your trapezius (large muscle extending from beside your neck down your back), rhomboids (muscles between your shoulder blades), and levator scapula (muscles above your shoulder blades).

Anterior muscles include serratus anterior (muscles between your upper ribs) and pectoralis minor (muscle beneath your pectoralis major).

All of these muscles make up your shoulder girdle. One of their purposes is to stabilize the scapula during activities such as push-ups.

Your glenohumeral shoulder joint is where the ball of the humerus (large bone in the upper arm) and the glenoid fossa (socket) of the scapula fit together.

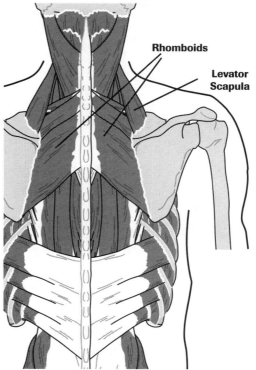

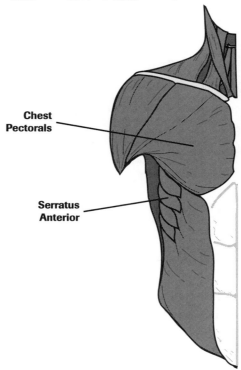

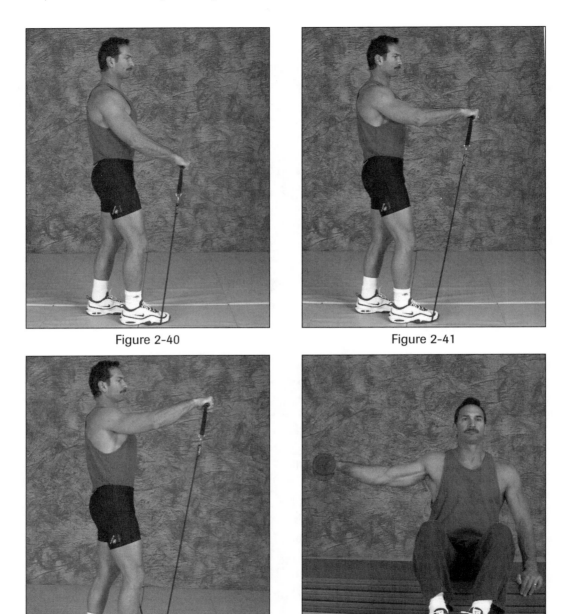

Figure 2-40

Figure 2-41

Figure 2-42

Figure 2-43

Flex your shoulder by lifting your arm up to the front in the sagittal plane. Extend your shoulder by bringing your arm back down. Abduct your shoulder by lifting your arm to the side in the frontal plane. Adduct your shoulder by returning it back toward your body (Figures 2-40 to 2-43).

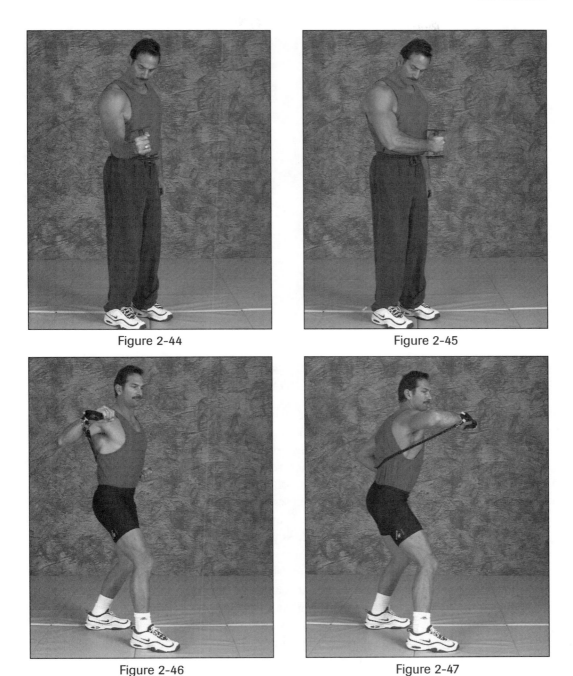

Figure 2-44

Figure 2-45

Figure 2-46

Figure 2-47

Externally rotate your shoulder by bending your elbow and taking it back as if to retract your arm to throw a hook punch (Figures 2-44 to 2-47). Internal rotation would be similar to a backfist strike. All of these movements take place in the horizontal plane.

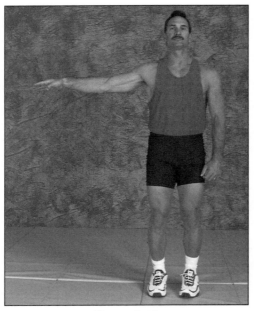

Figure 2-48

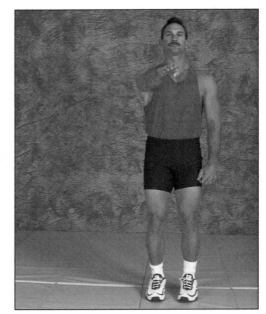

Figure 2-49

Horizontally flex your shoulder by extending your elbow and bringing your arm toward your body while keeping it at shoulder level (Figures 2-48 and 2-49). Horizontal extension is taking it back in the opposite direction.

The muscles of your glenohumeral joint include your deltoids, latissimus dorsi, and teres major. These muscles attach the humerus to the glenoid fossa of the scapula. They move the upper arm. Each of these muscles has a variety of functions depending on the angle of your arm. If you have pain in your shoulder when you perform push-ups, it may be because of tightness or weakness of these muscles, your shoulder girdle muscles, or your rotator cuff (supraspinatus, infraspinatus, teres minor, subscapularis) muscles.

Push-ups strengthen your triceps (back of your arms), pectoral muscles (chest), and anterior deltoids (front of your shoulders). To press your body away from the floor, extend your elbows by flexing your triceps. Horizontally flex your glenohumeral shoulder joint using your pectoralis major, anterior deltoid, coracobrachialis, and subscapularis. Your scapulae abduct (protract) using your pectoralis minor, serratus anterior, trapezius, and rhomboids.

When you perform push-ups, your head and neck remain neutrally aligned due to isometric contraction of your cervical spine. Abdominal muscles, erector spinae, and hip flexors stabilize your body to hold you in push-up position. Your abdominals are contracted to keep your lumbar spine (lower back) in neutral (slightly arched). And your hip flexors are contracted to prevent your hips from sinking to the floor.

See your doctor to rule out rotator cuff or impingement problems. Sixty percent of the power in your reverse punch may be funneled from your feet, through your hips, into your shoulder and out your wrist. Don't allow your shoulder to be your weak link.

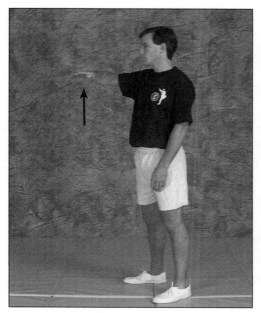

Figure 2-50

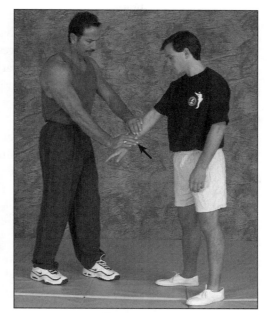

Figure 2-51

Figuring Out Shoulder Pain. Ask a dojo mate to watch your right shoulder blade (scapula) while you perform the following movement. Bend your right arm ninety degrees at the elbow. Slowly raise it (abduction). Continue to raise your arm without moving your shoulder blade (Figure 2-50). If you can lift your arm almost parallel to your shoulder without moving your shoulder blade, your rotator cuff may not be the problem. Also, if your collar bone (clavicle) were injured you could not raise your arm, period.

This time, let your friend provide light resistance as you lift your arm to the front (Figure 2-51). If you must tip your shoulder blade to avoid pain, you might have an impingement. The ball of your upper arm (humerus) might be bumping into the top of your shoulder socket (glenoid fossa). Or, there might be impingement of your fluid filled bursae sac. When the damaged bursae gets caught in the arch of your shoulder joint, it hurts. Your shoulder is reminding you not to raise your arm. It bulges when it becomes unhealthy. It may become thick and scarred with continued abuse.

Stage 1 symptoms of impingement syndrome include swelling and inflammation. You will feel tenderness in the shoulder joint, and pain and weakness with overhead blocks.

Stage 2 occurs when you have thickening of the subacromial bursae and tendinitis is apparent.

Stage 3 is evident with tears in the ligaments of the rotator cuff, tears in the biceps tendon, and changes in the bone. If you discover you have impingement syndrome, keep all blocks and punches below the level of your shoulder.

Your hip has a much deeper socket than your shoulder. Therefore, the ball and socket of your shoulder has less support than the ball and socket of your hip. Too much movement between the ball and socket of your shoulder may cause soft ligamentous tissue injury. This can lead to a subluxation where the ball moves around even more. A subluxation can generally heal without much intervention. A dislocation, where the ball comes completely out of the socket is serious, however.

Several ligaments provide a soft tissue barrier between your ball and socket. They limit motion, so when you cock your arm to throw a strike, your arm doesn't slide back out of your socket. These ligaments are as vital as your rotator muscles.

Your rotator cuff muscles hold the ball of your humerus in your shoulder socket as you extend your arm on your follow through. These muscles include your supraspinatus, infraspinatus, teres minor, and subscapularis. They should be strengthened. There are sever-

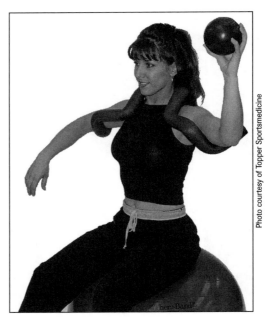

Figure 2-52

al simple exercises you can perform with light dumbbells or Sport Cords. Other devices maintain your form while you complete your rotator strengthening program (Figure 2-52). But some people don't train their rotators because they can't see them.

Pain has an inhibitory effect on your muscles. Muscles lose their connection when they are injured. Because the rotator cuff has a poor blood supply, damage to this area is slow to heal. If you injure your rotators, they may atrophy one hundred percent in a very short time because other muscles take over.

When you perform behind the neck shoulder presses, or lat pull downs, your rotator cuff muscles are in a shortened position. Shorter muscles are not as strong. They cannot stabilize the shoulder as well from this position. Perform most of your resistance exercises from slightly in front of your shoulder for greater strength and stability.

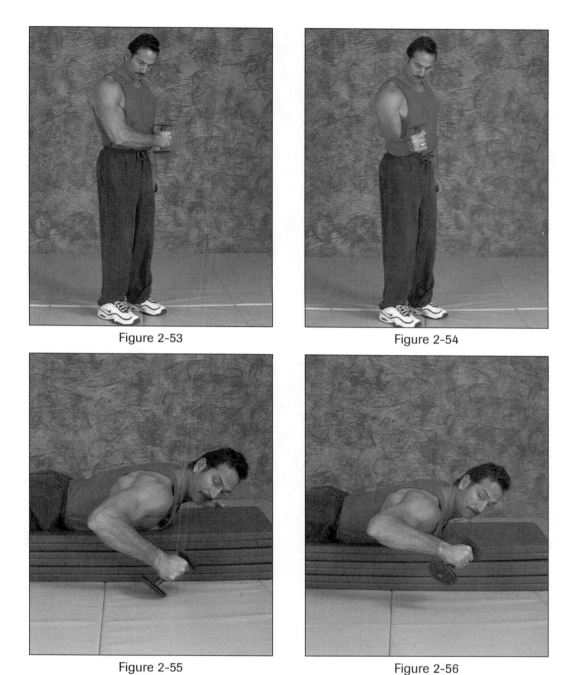

Figure 2-53   Figure 2-54

Figure 2-55   Figure 2-56

Ask your doctor or physical therapist how to perform the following exercises to fortify your shoulder for improved passing performance:
- External and internal rotation exercises (Figures 2-53 and 2-54).
- Reverse flyes in external rotation (Figures 2-55 and 2-56).

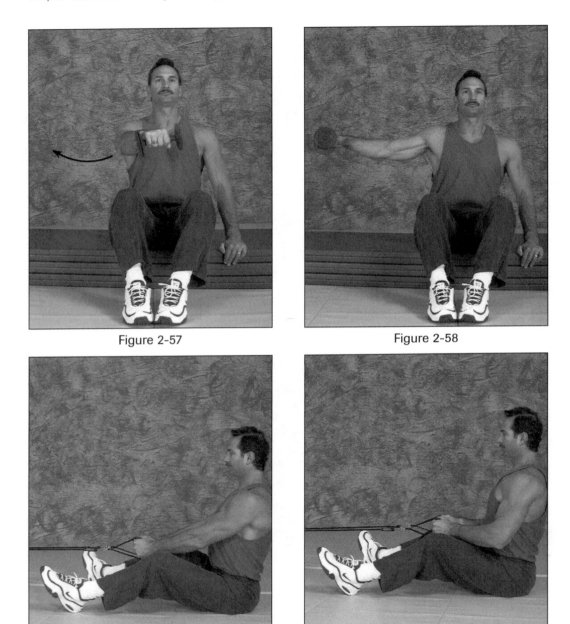

Figure 2-57

Figure 2-58

Figure 2-59

Figure 2-60

- Shoulder extension in external rotation (Figures 2-57 and 2-58).
- Rowing, lateral pull down (Figures 2-59 and 2-61).

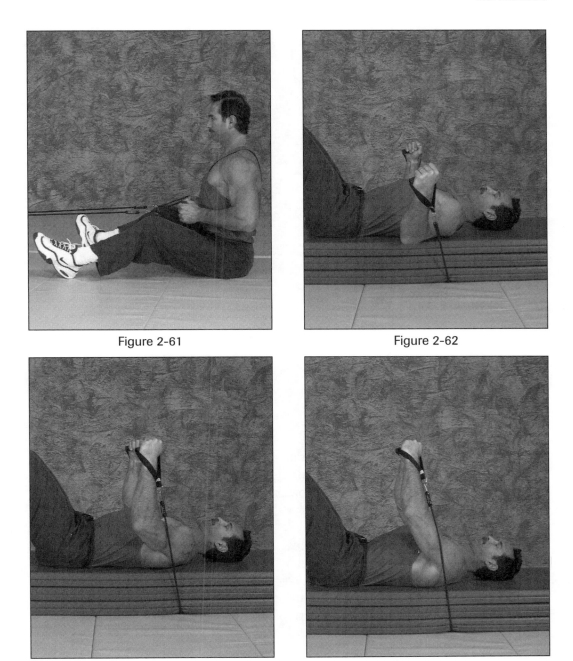

Figure 2-61

Figure 2-62

Figure 2-63

Figure 2-64

• Bench press with a limited range of motion (Figures 2-62 and 2-64).

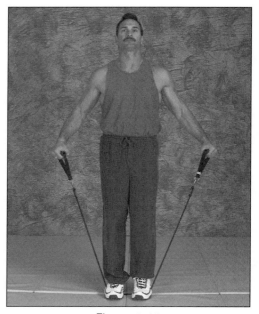

Figure 2-65

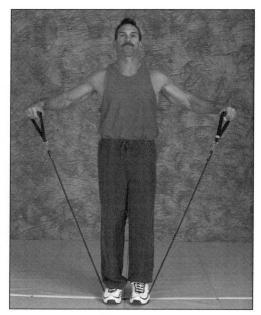

Figure 2-66

• Lateral raises (Figures 2-65 and 2-67).

Osteoarthritis

If you have pain in your joints when you practice martial arts, check with your doctor to find out if you have osteoarthritis. Osteoarthritis is a progressive, irreversible degeneration of the articular surfaces of the joints.

If you have arthritis you may have painful inflammation, swelling and limited range of motion in your joints.

Anti-inflammatories and analgesics are treatments of choice. Refrain from martial arts when your joints are inflamed. Focus on slow, Tai Chi range of motion and muscle strengthening. Since workouts may feel painful at first, try training just fifteen minutes, twice a day.

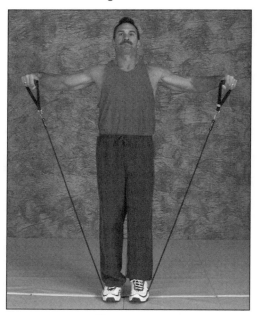

Figure 2-67

Women are affected more by osteoarthritis than men. And in older adults it is even more common. If you have problems climbing stairs and squatting, you might have osteoarthritis.

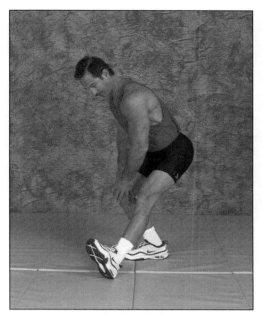

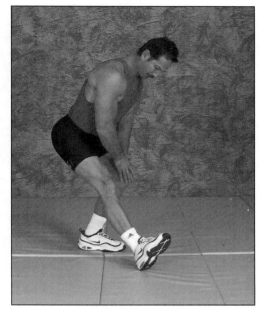

| Figure 2-68 | Figure 2-69 |

Jumping, running, and other high impact activities can be painful, and may worsen your condition. Especially if you compete in martial arts.

You might feel pain on the inside, outside, or middle of your knee. It can be localized or spread out. If your knees usually hurt when you practice martial arts, and they progressively get worse by the end of the day, you have symptoms of osteoarthritis.

Try performing your martial arts movements in a warm swimming pool. Practice your punches, kicks, strikes, and blocks against the resistance of the water. Do your katas in chest deep water. Any low impact activity is good. Avoid going up and down stairs and squatting.

If you are overweight, losing body fat can help take the load off of your joints. Your martial arts training should resemble Tai Chi in intensity, and always at an intensity below the level of pain. Be sure your exercise is regular. Try to follow an eating plan that keeps your body fat levels low to keep the stress off of your joints.

Tight hamstrings increase your osteoarthritis pain. Therefore your doctor may send you to a physical therapist to show you exercises to increase the strength and flexibility of your hamstrings and thighs. Your martial arts training has probably acquainted you with a variety of hamstring stretches, but here is an easy-to-do hamstring stretch that you can do anytime, anywhere.

Bend your right knee and place your hands on your right thigh for support. Extend your left leg forward with your heel on the floor and your toes pointed up. Gradually draw your hips back as you lengthen the hamstrings of your left leg. Switch legs and repeat (Figures 2-68 and 2-69).

To strengthen your thighs (quadriceps), practice your stances. But if you are too weak to hold your stances, begin with this exercise: sit on the floor with your legs extended to the

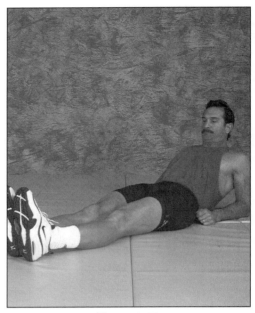

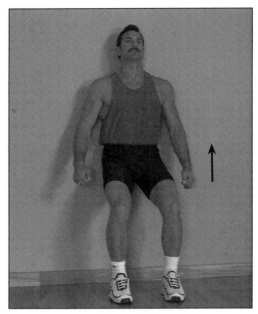

Figure 2-70   Figure 2-71

front and your hands behind you supporting your back. Slowly press the back of your knees toward the floor. Hold this position for three seconds, then relax. Perform ten repetitions of this exercise (Figure 2-70).

Another quadriceps strengthening exercise is as follows: lie on your back with your elbows supporting your upper shoulders. Bend your right knee so that your right foot is flat on the floor. Extend your left leg to the front and lift it a foot from the floor. Hold for ten seconds. Switch legs and repeat. Perform between ten to twenty repetitions with each leg depending on your level of fitness.

Wall slides will further strengthen your quadriceps. Sit against a wall with your knees bent. Lower yourself a few inches and hold that position for ten seconds. Slowly raise yourself to your original position (Figure 2-71).

If you have lost your meniscus or articular cartilage, it might be advisable to ask your doctor about an implant. Our present technology allows for transplantation, which helps to prevent any further negative consequences from the debilitating effects of osteoarthritis.

Osteoarthritis and the Knees. Randall Ideishi did not have an eight to five job like you and me. While we were sitting on our duffs, Randall was extending powerful kicks, and performing flips and jumps. Kicking to full extension, and jump kick landings caused swelling, pain, and a loss of motion in his knee.

Randall Ideishi, Taekwondo master and Olympic caliber (Ninja Turtle) superstar, found out the hard way he was human. In 1989 he went under the knife to repair his anterior cruciate ligament (ACL) and medial meniscus.

All was not well however. Scar tissue developed, and Randall was in a world of hurt. The medical term was arthrofibrosis—scar tissue in the knee joint. In 1992 Randall found his way to the world famous Steadman-Hawkins Clinic in Vail, Colorado. Dr. Steadman performed arthroscopic surgery to remove scar tissue, calcium deposit, or anything else that was not supposed to be there.

After the surgery, Randall was sent to renowned rehabilitation specialist, John Atkins, M.S., ATC., of the Topper Sportsmedicine Group in Vail. John, a Taekwondo black belt prescribed a variety of strengthening and stretching exercises for the muscles surrounding Randall's knee joint. A device called The Sport Cord was the only resistance equipment needed to provide the power his quadriceps and hamstring muscles required.

Atkins also prescribed a magic bullet. He suggested that Randall change the way he threw his kicks. Now if I approached Michael Jordan and told him I could improve his vertical jump he probably would walk, or run the other way. But John had a simple and direct cure for Randall's chronic knee pain—"Do not lock out on your kicks." John's exercise prescription and sage advice worked! Randall wisely followed John's program and walked away symptomless and pain free.

How many former martial artists do you know who quit because of knee problems? At best, they may have become world champions. At worst, they might have enjoyed the benefits of martial arts training for a lifetime. What if I were to tell you that if you hold back just a little on your kicks, you might practice martial arts into your twilight years? I'm not talking about kicking like a baby, simply do not extend your knee that last thirty degrees.

Atkins suggests that, "It is the responsibility of martial arts instructors to find out if their students have any pre-existing problems or injuries. Then they can go about setting goals and working around any physical difficulties." The philosophy of the Topper Sportsmedicine Group is to keep their patients safely in their sport. That same attention to safety exists at the Hansu Taekwondo School in Vail, where Atkins trains under the watchful eye of Dan Gnos. All ages and genders are exposed to the latest Sports-Medicine information on how to punch and kick for a lifetime.

Your knees are amazing joints. You stand on them all day long. But they are very much exposed. Knee joints are

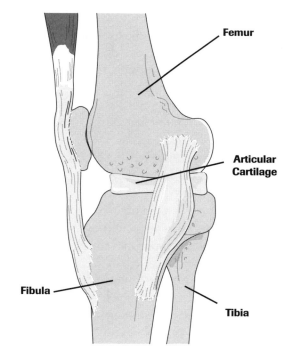

Femur

Articular
Cartilage

Fibula

Tibia

shallow, one bone does not fit tightly into another. Consider them similar to hinges. But when you bend your knees to ninety degrees, unlike a hinge, they can rotate too, making them even more complicated.

Your knee is your anatomical pulley between your femur (thigh bone) and tibia (shin bone) and fibula (small bone beside your tibia). Cartilage protects the ends of your bones and occupies the space between your bones. Consider cartilage as a cushion to prevent your bones from grinding. Your cartilage is filled with synovial fluid.

The end of your femur closest to your knee is enclosed by your femoral condyle. It is referred to as your articular cartilage. It protects the end of your femur. Aging can cause osteo-chondritis dessicans (cracks or fractures) in your articular cartilage.

You also have lateral and medial meniscus within your knee joint. These are cartilaginous material that have very little blood supply. They dry out with age and do not absorb as much fluid. Excessive rubbing of the end of the femur and tibia from full knee extension on your kicks may cause these cartilaginous fibers to wear out. Soon there is bone on bone contact. This is the origin of osteoarthritis.

Ligaments connect your bones together. Your lateral and medial collateral ligaments along with your anterior and posterior cruciate ligaments help to bring your femur in line with your tibia. Damage to your anterior cruciate ligament (ACL) may be a traumatic injury. Posterior cruciate ligament (PCL) impairment can also be severe.

Several muscles extend your knee. Your quadriceps allow you to extend your leg for a full force front kick. You can jump, and add power to your kicks using your extensors. These muscles (rectus femoris, vastus lateralis, vastus medialis, and vastus intermedius) are on the front of your thigh. The only one of these muscles that crosses your hip is your rectus femoris.

Your hamstrings, in the back of your upper leg generate knee flexion and hip extension. You use these muscles to pull down forcefully for your ax kick. And your hamstrings also help you to retract your front, side, roundhouse, hook, and back kicks. These muscles are gener-ally weaker than your quadriceps. If your hamstrings are more than three times weaker than your quadriceps, then you have a muscle imbalance which may precipitate knee problems. It is a good idea to strengthen your hamstrings (biceps femoris, semimembranosus, semitendi-nosus) using the Sport Cord.

On the inside of your knee closest to your groin, you have muscles called adductors. These muscles (adductor magnus, longus, brevis, and gracilis) help to pull your leg toward your body when you cock your kicks into a fold position. On the outside of your knee you have abductors. These muscles (tensor facia latae, gluteus medius) pull your leg away from your body when you perform roundhouse, side, and hook kicks. Your adductors and abduc-tors help to stabilize your movements when you flex and extend your knees from a standing position. There are a variety of known and unknown causes of knee pain. Tendinitis is gen-erally caused by overuse—jump kicks (especially landing).

Bursitis is irritation of the bursae sac in your knee. It may be caused by getting kicked in the knee or prolonged kneeling such as is required in your three minutes of meditation before and after class.

Ligament damage may be minor (1st degree) on a continuum to severe (3rd degree). Your ACL may be injured by twisting for your roundhouse kick and getting stuck in external rotation.

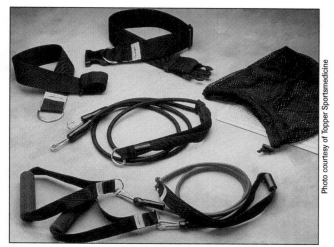

Your PCL may be damaged when you hyperextend your knee on a forceful thrust kick. But when your PCL is injured, usually this is accompanied by medial collateral ligament (MCL) or ACL strain. Your MCL and lateral collateral ligaments (LCL) may be damaged by a blow to the outside or inside of your knee, or knee rotation when your foot is planted.

Figure 2-72

Cartilage problems may be recognized by pain, clicking, or locking of your knee. But a loud "pop" is usually the ACL. Meniscal tears may be caused by a sudden twisting such as when a novice "ducks" too low trying to avoid a kick.

When you extend your knee, there is a slight lateral rotation of your tibia and femur. This is termed the "home screw mechanism." Some meniscus tears cause the knee to lock up because the torn meniscus gets caught in rotation.

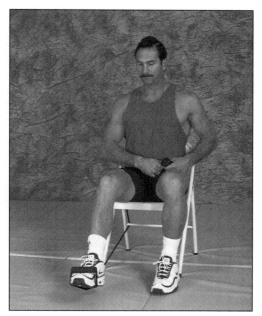

There is a 4:1 ratio of women to men who injure their ACL in martial arts. Possible explanations include weak hamstrings, poor conditioning, lack of pre-preparation agility drills such as plyometrics, and tracking problems in women because of their greater Q angle (wider angle from hip to knee).

Single leg, open chain exercises to strengthen the muscles surrounding your knees include leg extensions and leg curls using the Sport Cord (Figure 2-72). If your knees feel uncomfortable performing leg extensions, omit the last fifteen degrees of extension (Figures 2-73 to 2-76). In other words, don't lock out the knee at the top of the extension.

Figure 2-73

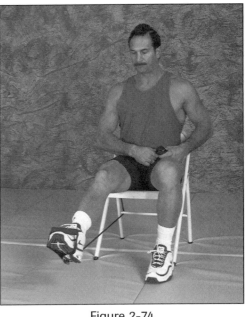

Figure 2-74

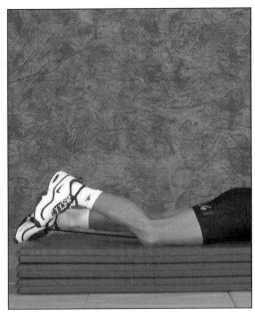

Figure 2-75

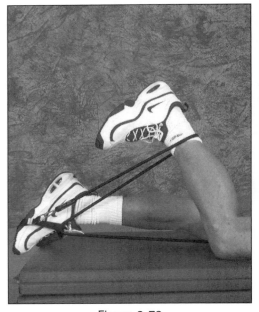

Figure 2-76

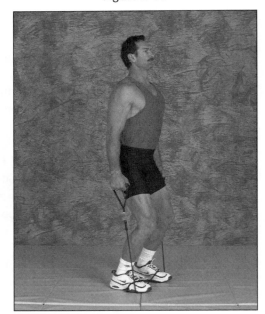

Figure 2-77

Double leg, closed chain exercises are closer to real world activity. These movements include half squats and lateral shuffling. Practice quarter squats, half-squats, and lateral and diagonal squats using the Sport Cord (Figures 2-77 to 2-81). Your physician can help you with these exercises.

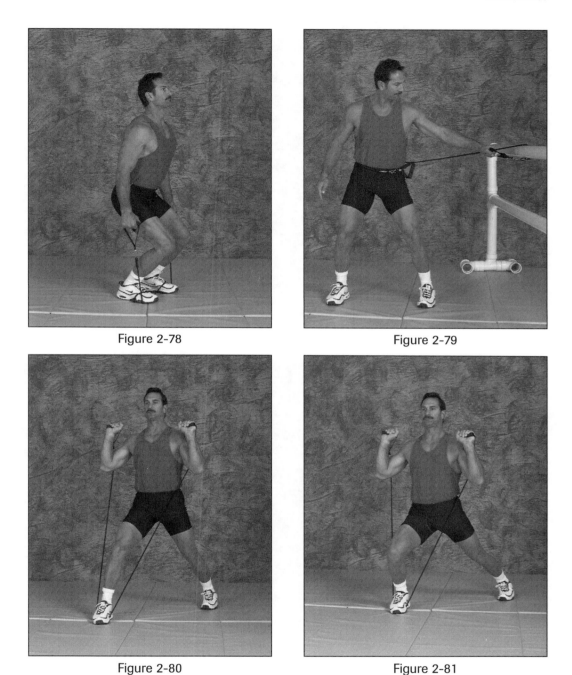

Figure 2-78

Figure 2-79

Figure 2-80

Figure 2-81

After mastering open chain and double leg closed chain exercises, try single leg closed chain activities. These include partial lunges, stationary lunges, and full translatory lunges. If you are successful with these, you may attempt diagonal lunges, and one-leg partial squats.

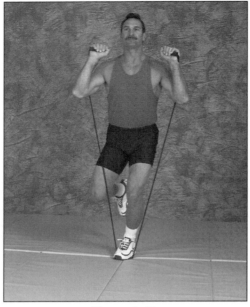

Figure 2-82

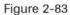

Figure 2-83

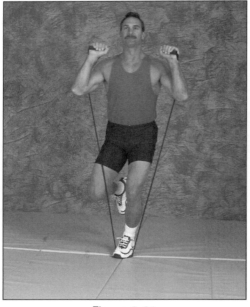

Figure 2-84

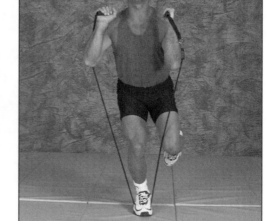

Figure 2-85

You may add resistance to all of these exercises with the Sport Cord (Figures 2-82 and 2-83).

When your muscles, tendons, and ligaments are strong enough, attempt to balance on one leg. Then close your eyes and continue (Figures 2-84 to 2-85). Find a balance board or wobble board to activate stabilizer muscles.

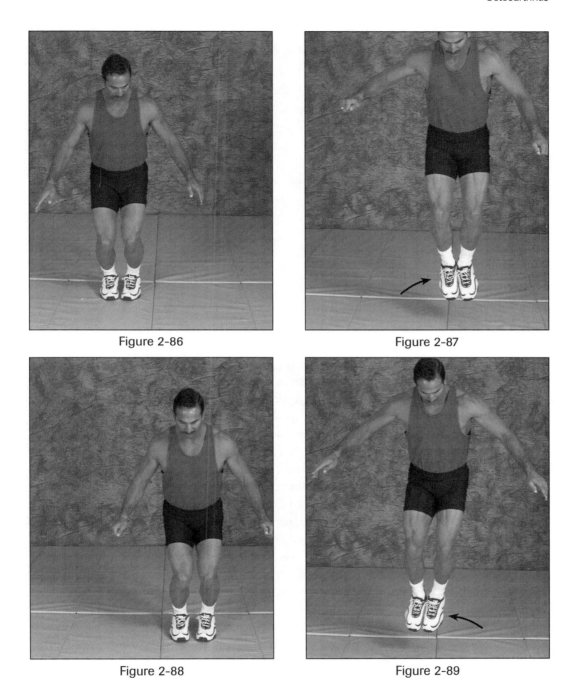

Figure 2-86

Figure 2-87

Figure 2-88

Figure 2-89

And if you are attempting to return to martial arts, try plyometrics. Plyometrics include forward, backward, lateral hops and leaps off both feet (Figures 2-86 to 2-89). Soon you may perform these same exercises with one leg.

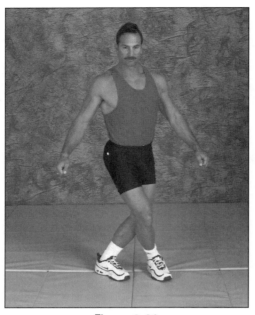

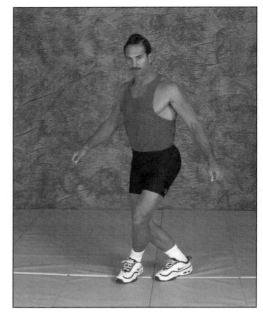

| Figure 2-90 | Figure 2-91 |

Progress to walk-jog-run-hop-jump drills (Figures 2-90 and 2-91). And when your knee is ready, agility drills and lateral movements such as the carioca and side shuffles are appropriate.

Your knees are supported by a variety of bones, cartilage, and ligaments. They are the anatomical pulleys connecting your thighs (quadriceps) and shins (tibia).

Talk to your doctor to rule out knee pathology. Chondromalacia is a progressive fissuring or softening of the patellar cartilage. Osgood-Schlatters disease is common in young teenage males where the bones grow faster than the muscles and there is irritation of the connection between the patella and the tibial tubercle.

Tendinitis and bursitis are uncommon in the quadriceps, but may occur in the musculotendinous junction high on the hip of the hamstrings. The iliotibial band, which stretches from the top of your hip to your knee, may become irritated by performing side, roundhouse, hook, and spinning kicks.

Patellar tendinitis may be caused by performing too many jump kicks. Within your knee joint is cartilage that protects the ends of the thigh bone (femur) and tibia. When you step down, you squish fluid out of cartilage. When you relax, fluid rushes back in. As you age, your cartilage does not absorb as much water. It dries out.

Ligaments save your joint when your opponent sweeps your leg. But if the outside (lateral) portion of your knee was hit hard, you may have "blown out" your lateral and medial collateral ligaments, and your anterior cruciate ligament.

Women sometimes have more trouble with their knees because of wide hips. The "Q" angle between their hips and knees is larger. A normal Q angle is ten degrees. If the Q angle exceeds ten degrees the knee cap (patella) becomes unstable. That is probably why you rarely see women with wide hips running marathons in the Olympics. Intense mileage for such events have selectively eliminated them from competition.

If your doctor performs surgery, you may find yourself in a cast or splint. Soon after your operation, you will be required to practice quad-setting, which is simply flexing your quadriceps for several seconds.

This is an isometric contraction used to prevent atrophy of the muscles surrounding your knees.

In addition, you will increase the range of motion (ROM) of your knees with stretching. Stretch all of the muscles in your legs from the ground up. Stationary cycling can help maintain your cardiovascular endurance while you increase the circulation in your legs. Sometimes your doctor may prescribe swimming with flippers (Figure 2-92) to increase muscular endurance.

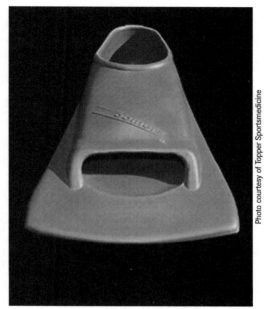

Figure 2-92

After your knees are rehabilitated, prepare yourself to begin a lifetime of strengthening and stretching exercises. Perform single leg open kinetic chain movements. Open chain activities allow you to isolate specific muscle groups without having to balance or stabilize them. To strengthen your quadriceps, sit on the edge of a table with your knees bent at ninety degrees. Hold a bucket on the top of your foot. Raise the bucket by extending your leg 180 degrees. Hold your leg straight for two seconds.

Slowly lower your leg to its original position for a count of four seconds. Add a few cups of water to the bucket each week until you can do ten repetitions with a bucket of water. Perform this exercise three times per week with both legs.

If you can get to a gym work your hamstrings using leg curls. Your quadriceps are generally stronger than your hamstrings. Leg curls may help prevent further muscle imbalance. Perform leg extensions (the bucket exercise) for your quadriceps with a limited ROM (terminal knee extensions) depending on your doctor's prescription. Then work the muscles on the inside of your thighs (adductors), and the muscles on the outside of your thighs (abductors) using a seated ad-abductor machine.

When your legs become stronger, begin double-leg closed kinetic chain exercises. These simulate movements in the real world. Start by sitting against a wall with your knees bent at ninety degrees. Slide up and down the wall strengthening your quadriceps and hamstrings (Figures 2-93 to 2-96). When you can comfortably perform ten repetitions of wall slides, step away from the wall and perform quarter and half squats. Be sure your knees do not extend over your toes. Execute half lunges and diagonal lunges to increase your balance. When your legs are strong enough, try one-legged half squats to prepare to return to martial arts.

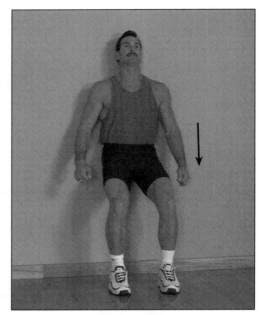

Figure 2-93

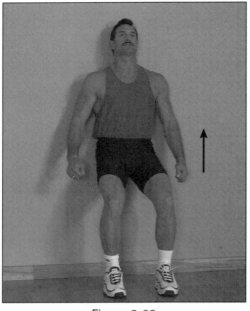

Figure 2-94

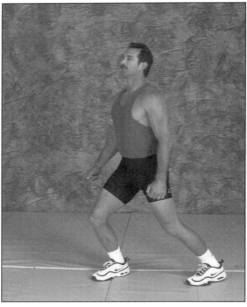

Figure 2-95

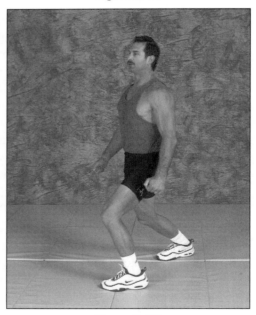

Figure 2-96

After your balance improves, challenge your neuromuscular system. The simple act of walking may be demanding. Between steps there is a momentary loss of balance. When walking becomes effortless, try standing on one leg like a stork or a flamingo (Figure 2-97). After you have mastered this stork pose, close your eyes and keep your balance on one leg for thirty seconds. Soon you may begin jogging, running, hopping, and jumping. When all of this is easy, experiment with agility drills or resistance training.

Anatomy of the Knee. The lateral collateral ligaments are on the outsides of your knees. Each connects your thigh bone (femur), to the small bone in your lower leg called your fibula.

On the inside of your knees you have your medial collateral ligaments. Each ligament links your femur to the large bone in your lower leg called your tibia.

Behind your knee cap (patella), two ligaments cross. The one typically injured is your anterior cruciate ligament (ACL). It connects your femur to your tibia. Your posterior cruciate ligament (PCL) unites these same bones.

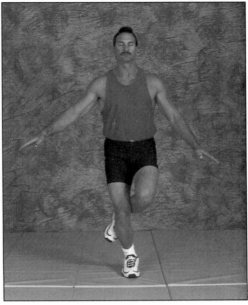

Figure 2-97

Ligaments attach one bone to another. They help to stabilize your knees. Consider them tent ropes. If one is slack it weakens the integrity of your entire knee joint. Your doctor may test for stability in each ligament by using manual manipulation.

Tendons join your muscles to your bones. They are strong, fibrous material. Tendons must be strengthened along with their muscular attachments, or they may weaken your power chain.

The tendons that bind your thigh muscles (quadriceps) to your knee joints are appropriately termed your quadriceps tendons.

Just below each knee, your patellar tendon joins your knee to your tibia. A tough, long tendon that extends down the side of your leg from your hip past your knee joint is your illiotibial band.

You have several sets of muscles that surround your knees. Your thigh muscles (quadriceps) are powerful and are located above and in front of your knees.

The purpose of each quadriceps muscle is to extend your knee upward for your front kick.

Your hamstrings are also very strong. They are located on the back of your upper legs. Your hamstrings flex your knees so you can pull-down for an ax kick. Knee flexion enables you return your leg as fast as you kicked.

Cartilage is the cushion between your bones. You have two semi-lunar cartilage (meniscus) in each knee that act as shock absorbers. These menisci are filled with synovial fluid. There is also articular cartilaginous material that protects the ends of your femur.

Other Causes of Knee Pain. Pain on the outside of your knee may be aggravated by friction on your iliotibial band. Stretching, anti-inflammatories, and ice may help.

Pain behind your kneecap may be Chondromalacia, a progressive softening of your patellar cartilage. Strengthen the quadriceps muscle on the inside of your knees by using the leg extension machine.

If you hold low stances, or didn't warm up properly you may have developed patellar tendonitis. Ice your patellar tendon for five minutes, massage it for five minutes, and then repeat this sequence.

Pain on the back of the inside of your knees may be bursitis. Three muscles, your sartorius, gracilus, and semitendinosis, meet at the pes anserine. Inflammation occurs at this site if these muscles rub against one another during ax kicks, and crescent kicks.

In any case, check with your doctor. She will probably ask for a more detailed history about the origin of your pain. She may also perform an arthrogram or arthroscopy to get a clearer picture of the reason for your distress.

Ankles

Ankles are the achilles heel of martial artists. In my dojo, no injuries are more common. An ankle sprain is generally a stretch or tear to a ligament. It may be a mild tear (grade 1), moderate tear (grade 2), or severe tear (grade 3).

Each sprain is a tear, it just varies in its degree of severity. Most sprains involve an injury to the ligaments on the outside of your ankle when your foot turns over. This is called an inversion sprain.

Sometimes you feel a "pop" where your ligaments are actually tearing. When your ligaments tear they bleed. This immediate bleeding increases inflammation beginning the extensive swelling that occurs.

If you injure your ankle answer the following questions:
- Did your ankle invert?
- What part of your ankle hurts?
- Was the pain so severe that your ligaments tore or your incurred a fracture?
- Could you stand up on it after the injury?
- Have you hurt this same ankle in the past?

R-I-C-E is the cure. "R" is for "Rest". Rest your ankle until you can walk without a limp.

"I" is for "Ice". Ice relieves pain and reduces swelling. Some of the chemical icings are too cold and can actually blister the skin. Pull a bag of frozen peas out of your freezer and ice your ankle for twenty minutes every two hours. Vegetable bags conform to the natural curve of your ankle. When your peas thaw out, grab a bag of corn. I use Dura Kold (Figure 2-98).

"C" is for "Compression". Compression, or a specially designed pressure wrap helps to decrease the swelling. Be sure to loosen an elastic wrap before bedtime. Physical therapists use a special machine called JOBST that sequentially squeezes the fluid from your foot and ankle.

"E" is for "Elevation". Holding your leg above your heart also reduces swelling. And at night, rest your ankle on a couple of pillows to keep your ankle above chest level.

Swelling is the body's way of cleaning up. The fluid is channeled through the lymphatic system. As the swelling subsides, you may notice a bruise. This is blood that is close to the skin. Sometimes, the degree of bruising is an indication of how badly the ligaments were torn.

The doctor's job is to determine what he must do to insure that the torn ligaments will repair themselves. He hopes that the ligaments overlap, and can be held in a neutral position until they heal. This sometimes requires a cast. Anti-inflammatory medication may help. Be sure to take anti-inflammatories with food. And some doctors recommend bracing until your ligaments heal.

A slow-healing sprain may not be a sprain at all. Often a slight fracture can cause less swelling than a sprain. An X-ray may help determine if you indeed have a fracture.

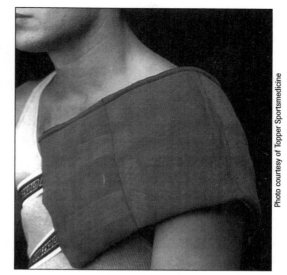

Figure 2-98

When you return to martial arts, practice balancing drills before you jump into plyometrics and sparring. Unused muscle and ligaments atrophy during your time away from martial arts.

Regaining your proprioception is your first priority to prevent another ankle injury. Proprioception is your ability to balance yourself. Simple exercises help your muscles and ligaments to stimulate nerve endings that were dormant during your recuperation. For example, stand on one foot while you perform your quadriceps stretch. Switch legs and repeat (Figure 2-99). Repeat these exercises again with your eyes closed.

Ankle problems do not necessarily require you to curtail your martial arts. Each case depends on the severity of the specific injury. You can return to your martial arts if you have a pain free normal range of motion. And be sure you can walk, jog, shuffle, and hop before you consider hardcore martial arts training.

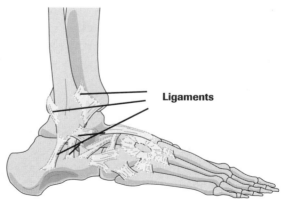

Ligaments

Stress Fractures. Shin-on-shin impact during sparring is a common martial arts injury. If you have pain in your lower leg, your training should be moderate and always at an intensity below the level of your symptoms.

Visit your doctor to find out exactly what your ailment is. You might have a stress fracture, compartment syndrome, tibial stress syndrome, or a sprain or strain. In any case the treatment depends on your diagnosis.

If the pain in the front of the bone on your lower leg (tibia) was sudden, you might have a fracture, bruise, tear, abrasion, or laceration. A gradual onset of pain however, may simply be overuse.

A sharp, focused, site of pain on the bone of your lower leg might indicate a stress fracture. Pain along the entire shin might be medial tibial stress syndrome a.k.a. "shin splints."

If your leg is pain free at rest, but hurts when you practice martial arts, or walk up and down stairs, you might have a stress fracture. Find a tuning fork and try this test. Pass a vibrating tuning fork along your tibia. If you feel a sharp pain, that indicates the possibility of a stress fracture at that site.

If your lower leg is painful at night however, even when you are resting, talk to your doctor immediately because these are symptoms of a tumor.

Stress fractures are caused by repeatedly overloading your tibia—sometimes by changing martial arts shoes or increasing your intensity. Take a look at your shoes. If they are more than six months old, and you train daily, they may have lost some resiliency.

Limiting impact is your first step to curing your stress fracture. Replace high impact plyometrics and bag work with shadow boxing and Tai Chi. If your injury is severe, a splint may be required.

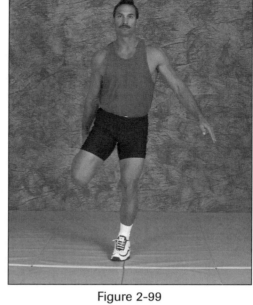

Figure 2-99

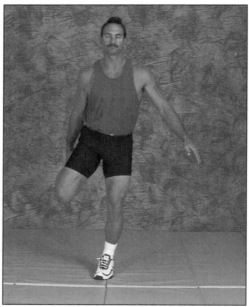

Figure 2-100

After your inflammation subsides and your doctor gives you the okay, try this exercise to strengthen the muscles on the front of your shins (tibialis anterior): walk on your heels with your toes up in the air for a minute (Figure 2-100). Add one minute a week until you can walk comfortably on your heels for three minutes.

Another strengthening exercise is to sit on the end of a leg curl machine. Place the top of your toes underneath the curling pad. Without moving your upper legs, raise your toes toward your knees (dorsiflexion). Do twenty repetitions with a very light weight three to four days a week. Always stretch both your calves and tibialis anterior after you complete these strengthening exercises (Figure 2-101 and 2-102).

Besides strengthening and stretching your lower leg muscles, research has demonstrated that females with menstrual irregularities, lower bone density, or less lean mass in the lower leg, are predisposed to incurring stress fractures.

If there is non-union of your tibial bone at the fracture site, and this is demonstrated by a black line on your X-ray, this fracture should be treated aggressively by a doctor. Usually a cast or immobilization is required. Sometimes a rod is inserted which would allow you to return to martial arts in six to eight weeks.

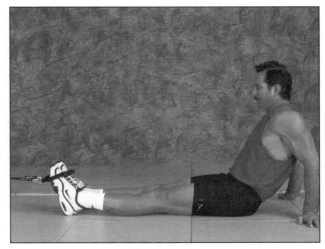

Figure 2-101

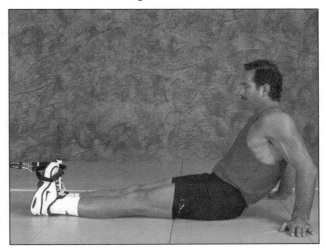

Figure 2-102

Blood

As you get older there is not as much oxygen rich blood to deliver nutrients to your working muscles for your punches and kicks. Aging causes blood vessels to become more rigid, restricting their ability to accept blood from the heart, resulting in high blood pressure.

Eating correctly, stress management, and exercise are the best conservative treatments for high blood pressure. A martial artist's blood vessels swell to twice the diameter of those of a sedentary person. Therefore, pressure is reduced, blood flow is increased, preventing a heart attack or reducing its severity.

Be sure to warm up and cool down with light shadow boxing for at least ten minutes. Monitor your blood pressure during your martial arts training. And keep your activity level low to moderate. Practice slow sparring and kata instead of fast.

Perform light repetitions on resistance equipment or the Sport Cord. Avoid pushing against an immovable object (isometrics) where you hold your breath (Valsalva Maneuver).

If you are on blood pressure medication (anti-hypertensives) such as ACE inhibitors, beta blockers, calcium channel blockers, or diuretics your heart rate will be altered. Do not rely on the heart rate formulas presented in this book if you are taking these medicines.

Your heart and blood circulation is a closed system. Liken it to a balloon half filled with water. If you add water or squeeze the balloon the pressure rises. The greater the pressure, the increased risk factors for coronary artery disease (CAD).

About thirty percent of martial artists have high blood pressure. And of those, seventy percent are classified as mild to moderately hypertensive.

High blood pressure exerts its impact in three primary organs. The heart (CHD), the brain (stroke) and the kidneys (renal failure).

Blood pressure is lowered by regular martial arts training. Several hours after a bout of exercise, blood pressure continues to lessen. Losing body fat may be a possible explanation for the profound effect exercise has on decreasing blood pressure.

This reduction may be the result of decreased fluid volume and or a decline in sympathetic nerve activity.

Abdominal Fat is Risky. Hopefully you have not let your ki drop to your waistline. Visceral fat in the abdomen is associated with metabolic disturbances that increase your risk of coronary heart disease (CHD). These disturbances include insulin resistance, glucose intolerance, hypertriglyceridemia, and reduced high density lipoprotein (HDL) cholesterol. You may lose weight faster from your waist but carrying excess weight in this area can be dangerous.

When you are nervous before a sparring match, the fight or flight response activates your sympathetic nervous system to prompt beta receptors to pull free fatty acids from your abdominal fat stores to be used for energy. Unfortunately, if you are predisposed to high cholesterol, a fatty buildup in your arteries may occur, increasing your chances for a blockage.

Dean Ornish, M.D., assistant clinical professor of medicine at the University of California, San Francisco, presented data demonstrating that a low-fat diet, stress management, and exercise form a non-surgical approach to combating heart disease, high blood pressure, and diabetes.

According to Ornish, it's easier to get a person to eat low-fat, exercise, and do stress management than to diet and exercise sporadically. His results showed that people who submerged themselves into an eating, exercise, and stress management program realized significant short term results, motivating them to continue for the long haul. Ornish's program includes less than ten percent fat in the diet (no saturated fat, so no animal products).

Diabetes. If you have diabetes, monitor your blood sugar frequently, eat properly, and continue your martial arts training. Participating in a regular martial arts training program may enable your doctor to reduce your medication. Be consistent in the frequency, intensity, and duration of your martial arts workouts to help stabilize your blood sugar.

If you are insulin dependent, and you are preparing to do a kicking routine, do not inject insulin into the working muscles of your leg. Be sure your blood sugar is above sixty before you exercise. Carry carbohydrate snacks during your activity. And monitor your feet for sores, abrasions, or blisters so you can provide immediate care.

Chronic Obstructive Pulmonary Disease. If you have chronic obstructive pulmonary disease (COPD) such as asthma, bronchitis, or emphysema certain precautions are necessary in order to continue practicing your martial art safely.

Maintain control of your breathing. Relax, take deep breaths from your diaphragm. Workout below the level of your symptoms. Vigorous sparring or kata may increase your breathing demand. Keep your inhaler available at all times.

Extend the time of your warm up and gradually increase your intensity. Accelerate the intensity of your martial arts workout no more than five percent during a single session. Drink water to avert dehydration. And avoid cold, pollution, and high pollen.

Muscles

Strength training must be an integral part of any martial arts program in order to achieve total-body health and fitness. You can dramatically improve the way you look, feel, and perform just by resistance training.

Training with weights or tubes improves your outward appearance and has far-reaching effects on your martial arts training. You'll be able to sculpt your body, improve your health, and enhance your punching and kicking performance.

When you add strength training to your martial arts workouts, you'll improve your cardiovascular fitness, muscular strength and endurance, body composition, and flexibility. Resistance training is your secret weapon for total fitness!

If you only have time for one form of exercise to round out your martial arts, weight training is the single best activity you can do for your body.

Your body loses about six pounds of muscle per decade. With less muscle your body burns fewer calories. You require less food, but if you eat the same as you did when you were younger you will gain fat.

Muscle is the engine for your metabolism. If you gain one pound of muscle, you must consume an extra fifty calories per hour to support it. On a brighter note, for every pound of muscle that you build, you can eat an extra fifty calories per hour without gaining fat.

Resistance training increases your bone density therefore decreasing your chances for osteoporosis. You will be stronger to rise from your stance or block a punch.

Maintaining muscle speeds up your metabolism and increases the good HDL cholesterol. More muscle helps raise your aerobic capacity and prevent type-II diabetes because additional muscle uses more oxygen, and takes up extra sugar.

You may or may not want to grow slabs of muscle like Arnold Scwarzenegger, but you can add to whatever muscle you have. Resistance training is the secret to strong, powerful attacks.

Check with your doctor. If everything is okay, begin strength training slowly. Fortunately, if you lifted weights previously, there is anecdotal evidence of muscle memory. Muscle memory implies that if you were muscular, it will be easier to restore. Specifically, you may have lifted weights in high school but not touched a weight since. You will increase your muscle sooner than someone who had never trained with weights will.

You may be forced to curtail your weight training due to an emergency or priority. But do not quit altogether. It is easier to maintain muscle then to regain it. And motivation to begin again may not come easy. A week's vacation is acceptable, but taking a month off means starting over. A prolonged break can lead to bone and muscle loss equivalent to several years of aging. Use it or lose it is a true phenomenon.

Lifting weights correctly never injured anyone. Problems arise when enthusiastic lifters try to hoist too much too soon. It is not how much weight you lift, it is how you lift the weight. Proper form is essential. Indeed, experienced lifters are not immune to injury. Lack of concentration, lackadaisical spotters, or equipment failure may contribute to injury.

Meso, Endo, or Ecto. A mesomorphic body type like Van Damme is one with well-defined muscles on the trunk and limbs. These folks are broader in the shoulders and hips and narrower at the waist. They have a high muscle to fat ratio and look fit even without weight training. Mesomorphs who lift weights notice a dramatic increase in strength and muscle mass.

An endomorphic body type is rounder, softer, and pear shaped. These folks appear to be aspiring sumo wrestlers. There is more fat surrounding their gluteals and thighs. Their muscles are not well-defined and they have a higher fat to muscle ratio. Resistance training helps with fat loss, but you must be patient. Tubing or weight training programs should focus on upper body development to balance endomorph's larger hip proportions.

An ectomorphic body type would look like Bruce Lee without muscles. Their bodies are long and rectangular, flat-chested, slender in the hips, with no defined waist. Ectomorphs have poor muscle development with relatively low body weight. This body type has difficulty retaining muscle. Ectomorphs must take in enough calories to balance their martial arts training caloric expenditure.

No matter which body type you possess, you will harvest the rewards of strength training: a leaner and stronger body. You'll see the improvement in your outward appearance, but more importantly, you'll also feel the difference.

It's no secret that a stronger body will improve your performance in your martial arts. If you are stronger, you can block better, and kick harder and faster without a second thought. Resistance training, specifically, will bring your overall martial arts skills to a new level. Resistance trained men and women generally have better reaction times, increased flexibility, endurance, and leaner body mass than non-lifters. This makes everything easier whether it's defending or attacking.

The American College of Sports Medicine (ACSM) recommends that strength training be an integral part of an adult fitness program. This is because weight training does not just produce cosmetic benefits, but delivers results you can feel as well as see. You can look forward to the following improvements in your health:

- Lower blood pressure
- Increase in food transit time through the colon to combat some types of cancer.
- Increased bone density, thereby decreasing your chance for osteoporosis.
- An increase in good HDL cholesterol.
- More muscle helps prevent type II diabetes because additional muscle uses more oxygen, and takes up extra sugar. Lower blood sugar levels are important for the prevention of type II diabetes.

How Strength Training Works. Strength training increases the size and number of the contractile proteins within your muscle fibers. Each muscle fiber is like an elongated cylinder that generally extends the length of the muscle.

Beneath the cell membrane or sarcolemma are the numerous thread-like structures that contain the contractile proteins of muscle. The thicker, darker, filaments are composed of myosin and the thinner, lighter filaments are composed of actin. Actin and myosin grow and proliferate. This in turn increases the size of the muscle fiber and its cross sectional area.

The motor neuron that transmits the electrical charge to the muscle has a distribution of mainly sodium ions located outside the neuron and potassium ions predominantly located inside the nerve giving the inside of the cell a less positive charge compared to the outside of the cell.

The axon that carries the impulse to muscles is blanketed with a lipid cover called a myelin sheath. Since neurons are composed of many nerve fibers, one function of this myelin sheath is to insulate impulses traveling along the same neuron.

It takes more than sixteen workouts to produce significant muscle fiber hypertrophy. The size and strength of connective tissue is increased which includes ligaments and tendons. There is an increase in the sarcoplasm (muscle cell fluid). High intensity strength training also increases bone mass and bone density.

You can enhance your muscular endurance by doing repetitions with resistance. The first phase of your improvement is due to neurological efficiency. You learn to recruit muscle fibers.

The second phase of your development is from strengthened connective tissue. Tendons and ligaments support your newfound muscle.

Muscle Fiber Type—Slow Twitch or Fast? The number of muscle fibers and type (fast twitch or slow twitch) in your body was determined during the 2nd trimester of your mother's pregnancy. Each of your muscle fibers is composed of seventy percent water, twenty percent protein, five percent phosphates, calcium, magnesium, sodium, potassium, chloride, fats, carbohydrates, and amino acids. You have 430 voluntary muscles which represents forty to fifty percent of your body weight. Skeletal muscle is the largest single tissue in your body.

You have two basic types of muscle fibers. Your postural muscles are Type I, endurance, red, and are considered slow twitch muscles. These muscles support your stances during kata and sparring. Type I fibers are recruited first during your strength and speed work and are capable of less force but can help you perform more repetitions (reps) and last longer in a marathon sparring match. Type I fibers utilize oxygen which means they are aerobic in nature. They are smaller and contain less glycogen than Type II fibers but their myoglobin content is high. They contain capillaries and provide endurance for a two hour non-stop kata class.

Type II, fast twitch fibers are recruited for fast, powerful punches and kicks. There are two subclasses of Type II fibers. Type II a-intermediate fibers are somewhat oxidative. They use a combination of the aerobic and glycogen systems. These are recruited after Type I fibers. Type II a-intermediate fibers are fast twitch with moderate myoglobin content, capillary density, force production and endurance. If you performed eight hard reps on the bench press, the first several reps utilized primarily Type I fibers. Next, Type II a-intermediate fibers assisted. And finally, when you were pushing out that last rep, Type II-b non-oxidative fibers were employed.

Type II-b fibers are non-oxidative (not aerobic). They are stronger and provide more force, but they fatigue quickly. Type II-b fibers are anaerobic with a high glycogen content and fast twitch rate. They have few capillaries and low endurance but a high power output for explosive attacks.

Muscle is Precious. Your muscles need glycogen, ATP, and innervation to become active. A stimulus to a motor unit contracts your muscles on an all-or-none principle. A muscle fiber will contract all the way, or not at all. One motor neuron may innervate one thousand muscle fibers in your quadriceps to execute a front kick, while another motor neuron may activate only ten muscle fibers to blink your eye.

Muscle takes up less space than fat. One pound of fat bulges eighteen percent more than a pound of muscle. Fat occupies 1.1 liters per pound while muscle requires just 0.9 liters per pound. Studies show that resistance training offsets any gains in circumference by losing fat. That is, if you do not increase your fat stores by wolfing down extra calories.

CHAPTER THREE

Strength Training

Strength training increases the frequency with which motor neurons are recruited and fired. Your golgi tendon organ senses an extreme stretch to a muscle. When your muscle is stretched to the point where the load you are trying to lift may be too heavy to handle, your golgi tendon organ forces your muscle to relax to prevent injury. The more you train with resistance, the less your golgi tendon organ kicks in. Some martial artists override their golgi tendon organs while yelling and screaming to hoist the weight up.

Biomechanical Sport Cord Resistance Training. Tubing is less expensive, less cumbersome, and takes up less space than weights. You can carry rubber tubing wherever you go, and gravity is unnecessary for its use.

Bands and tubes are made of synthetic materials such as carbon polymers, polyvinyl chloride, fiberglass, and rubber. As elastic stretches, the resistance increases.

In order for a resistance exercise to be effective, it must follow the line of pull of your muscle. When utilizing elastic resistance, the tube or band should fall in the same plane as the muscular action you are trying to challenge. The band should pull from the opposite direction of the muscular contraction.

When the band or tube reaches its elastic limit, the resistance increases dramatically and disproportionately. The same length of thicker tubing provides more resistance, but has less range of deformation before it reaches its elastic limit.

This decreases the available range of motion for a particular exercise and may cause too much stress on joints in certain positions. Using two tubes or bands increases the resistance similar to a thicker band and has the same range of deformation as a single band, therefore not restricting range of motion.

Place the band into the hinge of a door. This way, if someone opens the door, this is the last, not the first end to open. Always check the security of the attachment before performing any exercise.

Use hooks or wall mounted ballet bars as anchors. Hooks are placed in three different positions, approximately twelve inches from the floor, between your waist and shoulder, and one approximately six feet off the ground.

Tubing should be placed under the middle of your foot, and not under the toes as it can easily slip out and cause injury. Another safety tip—when performing exercises that require the band to be looped around your foot, loop it through your shoe laces too.

Check your band regularly for wear and tear. Look for changes in tension, splits, and cracks in both the tubing and the handles.

Study the photos closely to maintain perfect form on all of your exercises. Gradually increase your intensity until you reach your desired strength, flexibility, and endurance goals.

Warm Up. The purpose of your warm up is to prepare you physically and mentally for your Sport Cord resistance workout. Begin walking or jogging at an easy pace using your belted Sport Cord resistance attachment. Your body temperature increases, getting you "fired up" for your training.

Short Term Goal. During the warm up, imagine yourself performing each Sport Cord resistance exercise, step by step, and with perfect form.

Long Term Goal. During the warm up, "see" and "feel" your long-term martial arts performance goals.

Sport Cord Stretching. Your Sport Cord pre-stretches your muscles prior to each exercise. But we recommend you perform an additional full body stretch prior to your Sport Cord resistance-training workout. Be sure your muscles are sufficiently warm before you begin stretching. Exhale into each stretch. And relax through the full range of motion as demonstrated in your text. Stretching prevents injury, lubricates your joints, and increases your coordination and mobility.

Doctor. Consult your physician if you are over forty years old, or have a pre-existing medical condition before you begin exercising with the Sport Cord. Address any joint pain or unusual aches with your physical therapist or doctor immediately. This will provide peace of mind so you may enjoy your workout. And if your doctor has a few moments, demonstrate your favorite Sport Cord exercises. Maybe you can convince your doctor to join you on your Sport Cord adventures.

Metabolism—Yin/Yang. One-third of martial artists are currently overweight. Just fifteen years ago, only twenty-five percent were overweight. This is an increase of thirty-two percent. The average adult martial artist weighs eight pounds more now than ten years ago.

Natural weight or "ideal" weight can be described as the weight at which your body comfortably stays while eating for appetite and practicing martial arts regularly. Primitive folks burned approximately 2,900 calories per day hunting and gathering food. Today the average American burns only 1,800 calories.

If both of your parents are obese, you have an eighty percent likelihood of becoming obese. If one of your parents is obese, there is a forty percent probability that you would be obese. If both of your parents are lean however, there is only a fifteen percent chance that you will weigh more than twenty percent over your ideal weight.

A study on identical twins indicated that genetics plays a critical role in what they weigh. Identical twins separated at birth weighed nearly the same after years of living apart.

Another interesting study was done on twins by researcher Claude Bouchard. Results showed similar weight gains among sets of identical twins when they were fed one thousand extra calories daily for 120 days. A fascinating outcome was the wide variance of weight gain between the sets of twins. Some sets gained as little as eight pounds with the over feeding while others ballooned up as much as twenty-nine pounds. Clearly this demonstrated that genetics play a major role in weight gain. But this investigation also demonstrated that there are other influences that determine weight. Some people gain more and others less, with the same stimulus.

Between the ages of thirty and seventy, it is estimated that your fat free mass (muscle) declines by forty percent. This is thought to be the single most important reason why you store more body fat as you age. The loss of fat free mass and resulting slow down of metabolic rate makes you susceptible to gaining fat. Each pound of lean tissue burns approximately fifty calories a day. A loss of just half a pound of muscle or twenty-five calories expended daily, could theoretically cause you to gain 2.6 pounds in a year. In ten years, twenty-six pounds. In twenty years, fifty-two pounds. In thirty years, seventy-eight pounds.

There are three critical times when you gain fat cells:
1. The last trimester in the womb.
2. The first year of life.
3. During puberty.

When you gain weight you increase the size of your fat cells. When you lose weight, you decrease the size of your fat cells. Normal cell size is 0.5–0.6 micrograms. The upper limit is 1.0 micrograms. When fat cells are full, your body can make new ones. However, when you lose weight, the fat cells do not disappear. Therefore, if your training partner has more fat cells than you do, he will ultimately be fatter as each of those cells will contain some fat.

Your body is not physiologically designed to lose weight or fat rapidly. One pound of fat supplies the energy to walk nearly thirty miles. Your body uses about fifty percent fat and fifty percent carbohydrate at rest. During martial arts training this will change, depending on your intensity. At high intensity sparring, you use a greater percentage of carbohydrates. At lower intensities, a higher percentage of fat is used. Alternating high and low intensity intervals is a tremendous advantages for weight loss and weight control. You should not be concerned with which fuel you are burning at the moment, but rather how many calories you are expending during and after your martial arts training.

To receive the greatest value from your martial arts training, strive to become as fit as you can so you burn more calories from fat at rest, and utilize more storage fat during your training.

It is better to be disciplined about your eating than fanatical. Fueling your muscle is a major part of your martial arts success. What you eat today and tomorrow will benefit your martial arts the next day, and the next.

Your bones and muscles require high density micro nutrients from foods you eat. Trace elements and iron are needed to rush oxygen to your working muscles. High quality proteins are essential to maintain your strength. And adequate minerals and water are necessary to sustain your electrolyte balance.

You may burn between 300 to 500 calories per martial arts workout. Therefore, be sure you are consuming enough food. Your first step is to eat a combination of carbohydrates (starches) and protein (lean meat or dairy) for breakfast. A sandwich-snack between breakfast and lunch helps stabilize your blood sugar. Have a hearty lunch to fuel your afternoon martial arts workout. And, refuel after your workout. This seems like a lot of food. Initially, you may have difficulty reminding yourself to eat. Soon you will anticipate each meal, and snack. Balancing your meals energizes your punches and kicks.

There are no junk foods or pure health foods on your eating program. Depending on your age, gender, and martial arts goals, match foods to your needs. Obviously, there is no magic formula that works for everyone. Your goals are unique, and so is your body.

You burn carbohydrates, proteins, and fats. If you were training for the World Championships you would eat more carbohydrates than if you train twice a week and on an occasional weekend. Depending on your total caloric expenditure and exercise intensity, balance your caloric intake accordingly.

Experts agree that at least half of your calories should come from carbohydrates, no matter how active or inactive you are. If you take in less than fifty percent carbohydrates, your fat intake rises incrementally. And increased fat is unhealthy. Martial arts performance diminishes when less than fifty percent of your calories are from carbohydrates.

You can guesstimate your total carbohydrate need by your energy levels and how your weight changes over the course of a week. A suggested formula to estimate your carbohydrate intake per day is to multiply eight by your weight in kilograms. Or, visit a health center to discover your resting metabolism. Your resting metabolic rate is how many calories your body burns at rest. You metabolize foods differently now than when you were a teenager. And in your older adult years, your metabolism will change again.

Nutrition

Martial arts training is easier when you stoke your muscles for workouts. Carbohydrates and protein energize you for peak martial arts performance. Eat and drink correctly and use a variety of mid-meal snacks to fill in the gaps. Protein milkshakes, energy bars, and energy gels are in vogue. But supplements are not to be taken in place of food. Consume them in addition to, not in replacement of, a well balanced eating program.

As recent as a decade ago martial artists relied heavily on information passed down from competitor to competitor. To lose bodyfat it was suggested to guzzle soft drinks. We were told, "They burn up the fat." For breakfast we were advised to eat a concoction of raw egg and ginseng. Sometimes water was withheld during strenuous workouts to toughen us.

Most Americans eat red meat, chicken, turkey, pork, potatoes, salads, fruits, rice, beans, peas, and grains. Lean folks eat the same foods, they merely prepare them differently. They choose round steak instead of hamburger, chicken and turkey breasts instead of dark meat, pork loin instead of bacon, baked potatoes, rice, and beans, instead of french fries, fried rice, and refried beans. They trim the fat and bake, broil, and grill rather than fry. Low fat does not mean dry, baked potatoes and tasteless, cottage cheese. Low fat, low calorie can be as appetizing as turkey burgers and baked fries. It is in the preparation. Substitute applesauce, non fat cremes, and egg whites for high fat items such as oils, creams, and egg yolks. Create non fat delicacies that taste like the real thing. Choose low fat over high fat and you should lose inches.

But we do need some fat. We should eat between fifteen and twenty-five percent fat. For men that is about sixty grams of fat on a 2,500 calorie diet. And women should take in about forty grams of fat on a 2,000 calorie diet. Your activity level helps determine the amount of calories and fat to consume. The more you exert the more food you need.

Your final step is to respect healthy routines and end bad patterns. No more dieting. Remember the last time you dieted? You gave up all of your favorite foods. Then after a month, you were blindsided by a pizza commercial. You decided to eat just one slice of pepperoni pizza and save the leftovers. The last thing you remembered was devouring the entire pizza and thinking, "I blew it so I might as well indulge in a carton of ice cream." And you proceeded on a Blue Bell frenzy. Days later your gi pants were tight. You fell off the wagon, gained all your weight back, and a few pounds more. The same foods you abandoned when you started your diet were the ones that precipitated a binge. You thought it was your fault that you couldn't resist cravings. You blamed it on lack of willpower. But you didn't fail. Your diet failed you.

It is less painful and more fun to train in martial arts, drink water, and eat low fat. But if you cannot eat just one, don't. Whether you are addicted to chocolate, chips, or you just love to binge, don't give in.

Examine your schedule. Figure out when you get hungry. Have appropriate snacks available such as bagels, fig bars, Graham crackers, fruit, energy bars, pretzels, non-fat yogurt, and non-fat popcorn.

Beware of celebrating or drowning your sorrow in edibles. A recent study in the February issue of the *American Journal of Clinical Nutrition* concluded that stomachs actually stretch after a humongous meal. Dr. Allan Geliebter suggests, "Packing in huge amounts of food in one sitting is the culprit. Many overweight martial artists skip breakfast and have a very small lunch. That's probably not enough time to shrink stomach capacity. And, by the time dinner rolls around, they're ravenously hungry and swallow huge volumes of food. Night after night following this eating routine might eventually increase stomach capacity. The now-larger stomach requires more food to feel full."

Strive to keep your blood sugar level. Consume several small mini-meals throughout the day. Feed your muscle. Starve the fat. Stay on a tolerable eating and exercise program all of the time rather than depriving yourself, and then doing a food fling. Be patient. You lose fat in ounces not pounds. Develop healthy habits and soon you won't obsess about food.

Decide the hours during the day when are normally hungry. If you don't know what it feels like to be hungry, symptoms include feelings of listlessness and fatigue. Your blood sugar may drop.

Food provides energy. Most of us need an energy boost every couple of hours. Choose morsels that feed your muscle. Eat and drink just enough to satisfy. Substitute your normal high fat/calorie fare for low fat/calorie items.

Fad diets don't work. Temporary weight loss programs provide temporary results. It's easy to follow a step-by-step plan of cabbage or grapefruit and lose weight. The weight you lose is fat, muscle, and water; probably not in that order. When you return to a semblance of your normal eating pattern you will gain your weight back, and more.

Rather than deprive yourself, eat sensibly. The single most important feat you can accomplish to insure you will lose body fat is to eat a healthy breakfast. A good choice is oatmeal, non fat milk, and a banana or raisins. Carry a cooler in your car filled with plastic containers of your favorite non-fat foods. Turkey sandwiches, non-fat yogurt, sliced vegetables, fruits, and low-sugared drinks are some easy choices. If you get hungry between breakfast and lunch choose non-fat yogurt. Enjoy a sandwich for lunch along with sliced fruit. You may be too busy between lunch and dinner for a full-blown snack. Mix a meal replacement product for a one-minute delicious shake. Dinner should be fun. Create low fat cuisine substituting high-fat with low-fat items.

You Know What To Do, Do It! Losing weight does not require willpower—what you need is information. Ninety-five percent of those who attempt a low calorie diet gain their weight back, and more. Healthy foods such as fruits, pasta, cereal, bread, olive oil, peanuts, and peanut butter are not necessarily useful in your weight loss program.

Martial artists cut calories and increase their activity too much, slowing their metabolism. Their energy levels drop and their bodies conserve fat. Instead of fueling their muscles throughout the day, most martial artists backload. They eat late in the day. This helps to conserve fat. Excuses include no time or money. It is in fact less expensive to pre-prepare foods in plastic containers rather than rushing to a fast food establishment and paying several dollars for a baked potato.

Other Diets. Everyone is looking for a quick fix when it comes to diet. Fad-fraud programs promise rapid weight loss, but they do not work. They usually lack carbohydrates, which leads to muscle and liver glycogen depletion.

Since water is stored with carbohydrates (breads, pasta, potatoes, rice, etc.), when you stop eating carbohydrates, you notice a rapid water weight loss. This looks and feels okay at first, but in a short time, water weight returns. The bad news is you did not lose an ounce of fat. And when your water weight returns, your resolve diminishes.

It is not surprising you felt a lack of vigor on your diet. You probably were irritable too. Carbohydrates are your muscle's best source of energy, similar to rocket fuel for your muscles. Low-carbohydrate diets frustrate your ability to exercise because your muscle glycogen stores are drained.

These diets encourage low blood sugar (hypoglycemia) because your liver glycogen stores are spent. When fats and proteins are broken down to be used for energy you may feel sluggish. Instead of burning carbohydrates for energy, your body used fat and protein (ketosis), causing symptoms such as nausea, loss of coordination, and an inability to concentrate. Besides, taking in less carbohydrates usually means stocking up on fats which increases your risk for heart disease.

The Zone Diet, created by Barry Sears, is based on the belief that eating carbohydrates raises insulin so your body will store more fat. Selected studies suggested that when diabetics injected too much insulin, they gained fat. And it is true that high glycemic foods (foods high in simple sugar) tend to raise insulin levels. But it is also true that high glycemic foods generally have more calories.

Grinding and mashing foods increases glycemic index (GI) by speeding digestion and sugar utilization. GI is measured by how fast the carbohydrate you consumed is converted to blood sugar. Apple juice has a higher GI than the apple from which it was squeezed. The fiber and larger apple particles take longer to be assimilated than a cup of apple juice that finds its way quickly to the bloodstream. Below are some foods and their glycemic index.

Foods	Glycemic Index (GI)
Honey	87
New potato	70
Brown rice	66
Oatmeal	49
Whole wheat spaghetti	42
Orange	40
Apple	39

Any excess calories not used for energy will be stored as fat. But compared to fat, carbohydrates are more likely to be used for energy. Barry Sears suggests that to burn body fat more readily, you should eat forty percent carbohydrates, thirty percent protein, and thirty percent fat at each feeding throughout the day. His theory is that if you eat more fat, you will burn more fat.

Carbohydrates and Protein. The authors of several new books including *Healthy For Life, Enter the Zone,* and *Protein Power* suggest high protein should replace carbohydrates in your diet to lose fat. Their assumption is that carbohydrates increase insulin, which causes your body to store fat.

But insulin is a good thing. Insulin carries nutrients from your blood stream into your cells. Insulin is the vehicle that provides your muscles with energy.

Carbohydrates don't make you fat, calories do. If you eat more calories than you burn, you gain fat. Excesses of carbohydrates, proteins, or fats can leave you with an unwanted spare tire. The lesson here is that carbohydrates are not the enemy, and that we need a balance of fuel substrates for maximum performance. Therefore, any diet program that recommends less than fifty percent carbohydrates, is doomed to failure.

Several factors determine how many calories you expend. If you are bigger, you dissipate more calories than a smaller person. The harder you work, the more calories you disperse. If it is extremely cold or hot, your body burns extra calories to maintain your normal temperature. And if you are fit, you fritter away more calories than a sedentary person, even in your sleep.

The "low fat" craze gave you an excuse to overdose on sugar. Although you, and most Americans, now eat less fat and more Snackwells, everyone is fatter than ever.

Fasting. Some people fast for religious reasons, others to "cleanse" their bodies, and still others to lose fat. Fasting to lose fat is a fantasy. When you eat less than a few hundred calories a day, you lose water, muscle, and a little fat. This slows your metabolism and depletes your liver and muscle glycogen. Seven days of fasting can cause you to lose a third of your muscle.

You have little energy for martial arts training, and even if you did, you would be burning precious muscle tissue. In addition, fasting for more than a week can cause mineral imbalances, low blood pressure, kidney stones, impaired kidney and liver function, and anemia. And when you gain your weight back, you will be fatter than ever.

Vegetarianism is becoming popular because many people believe meat is bad for your health. And it is, if you eat meat that is high in saturated fat. Turkey, chicken, egg whites, lean cuts of beef, pork, and lamb can provide you with a significant source of lean, high quality protein. You need protein daily so try to include lean sources of protein in a carbohydrate base.

Fast food restaurants sell lean roast beef sandwiches. But beware of too many hamburgers. Even if you purchase ninety percent lean ground beef from your grocery store, fifty percent of those calories are from fat. To reduce the fat, brown your ground beef, throw it in a colander and rinse it in hot water. After rinsing, place the meat back into a clean pan. Use it sparingly, as an ingredient in tomato sauce and other recipes.

Meat is an excellent source of iron, zinc, and B vitamins. As a vegetarian, you can get iron, zinc, and B vitamins from plants, but they are not as readily absorbed. If your lack of energy stems from anemia, eating red meat a few times a week can give you a boost. The darker the meat, the more iron available.

Be careful not to succumb to tempting, quick fix, devices such as rubber suits, sauna wraps, or thigh cremes. At best these provide you with temporary water loss to "feel" smaller. But once you drink water, back comes the weight. Nonprescription herbal diet pills vary in potency and may be dangerous. Ephedrine based products can induce rapid pulse, arrhythmias, and in a few cases, death.

Diabetic Diet. If you are a diabetic, don't skip meals. If you miss breakfast you might incur low blood sugar. Your body falls into a starvation mode. You may be irritable and your energy drops. When you finally eat, you may devour too much. Spread your meals into manageable feedings about every three hours. Tastes can be changed and habits altered by making low sugar choices in several small meals through the day.

Eating frequently is an effective plan for an infant, child, martial artist, and diabetic. A study in *The New England Journal Of Medicine* showed that over a three week period a group of men ate three meals a day totaling about three thousand calories. Several weeks later they again ate three thousand calories each day, but this time they dispersed their meals into seventeen small ones. Their food was absorbed more efficiently, and the nutrients were utilized more effectively when they were grazing throughout the day. In addition, their metabolic rates increased and so did their energy levels. Eat six small meals a day and in three weeks you may lose your rumbling stomach, be less irritable, and have increased energy.

Develop a healthy lifestyle with exercise and eating. Choose foods your body needs, not what some television commercial fools you into believing. It is easy to become addicted to high sugar foods that have little nutritional value. Baked chicken, tuna, brown rice, and potatoes may not compare to ice cream, candy bars, and cotton candy until you begin to listen to your body.

In one study, subjects were permitted to choose from a variety of fruits, vegetables, meats, cakes, and ice cream. At first most chose desserts, but within weeks they craved fruits and vegetables.

Most of us grab something quick on the way out the door such as peanut butter and jelly on processed white bread with a bag of chips. Dinner is often microwaved from the freezer. Snacks are sugar-laden juice boxes and white flour crackers. And we expect to lose weight.

Eating wholesome food requires preparation. One solution is to pre-prepare nourishing foods. Fill plastic bags with nutritious sandwiches, dry cereal, graham crackers, and a variety of ready to eat fruits and vegetables. Preparing edibles in advance ensures that food is always on hand so low blood sugar won't trigger visions of candy bars and ice cream.

Nutritionist Keith Klein advises us to make better bad choices. Instead of storing ice cream in the freezer, purchase individual servings of sugar-free frozen yogurt. Rather than squandering carbohydrates on a single cookie, enjoy a hefty bowl of sugar-free pudding. If you crave a candy bar, increase your dose of regular insulin according to your physicians recommendations.

Another trick is to phone in a special-order to your favorite restaurant. If your blood sugar is high, give your injection at home and by the time you arrive your dinner will be ready. You will need to be prepared for low blood sugar if dinner is late by carrying crackers or juice to tide you over. Ask that your foods be prepared without additional sugar. Dressings and sauces can be ordered on the side to regulate carbohydrates. Your waitperson may more readily heed your special order if you explain that you are diabetic.

You must individualize your eating to your martial arts. When you increase the frequency, intensity, or duration of your workouts, add extra carbohydrates to your pre- and post-workout meals or decrease insulin with your physician's advice. You might try about fifty supplementary carbohydrates for each hour you plan to exercise. Your energy level soars when you preserves your muscle glycogen stores through systematic snacking. If you fail to increase your carbohydrates your blood sugar plummets and you may feel droopy. You may feel weak or uncoordinated when carbohydrate sources are low leading to possible injury. You need fuel for repair and to provide nourishment.

Your thirst mechanism may malfunction during your martial arts training. Bodyweight may drop a few pounds before feeling thirsty. You may dehydrate or experience hypoglycemia during a workout. When you work out, your blood sugar generally decreases. To prevent this sip carbohydrate juices or sports drinks between exercises. Carbohydrate sports drinks and juices are quick energy. Look for sports drinks with between ten and twenty grams of carbohydrates per eight ounce serving. Sometimes they are too sugary, so you may dilute them with water. Make sure your drink has equal amounts of potassium and sodium (about fifty milligrams in an eight ounce serving). A variety of sports drinks are on the market. Be sure you enjoy the taste (you will drink it if you like it).

Cereals are a quick, convenient, nutritious and delicious way to add carbohydrates to your food plan. Eat fortified cereals that are high in fiber and vitamins. Shredded Wheat contains zero grams of refined sugar and is nutrient dense. Add an artificial sweetener for taste. Sugar Smacks, Cap'n Crunch, and Frosted Flakes contain between thirteen and fifteen grams of empty sugar calories. Keep track of the total number carbohydrates. Most nutritionists recommend any food less than twenty calories is free.

Eating for Health and Fitness. Some martial artists have not developed coping skills to handle stress. Although they teach a variety of mind/body techniques, they are not task oriented. Instead, they hide from their problems by eating.

Others have not learned to view themselves in a positive way. Over-eating makes them feel better. They may also view themselves as failures when they cannot succeed at weight management.

Stress is a major cause of relapse. Tackle your problems rather than eat. Recognize situations over which you have no control, and learn to let them go. Over-eating does not solve problems, it creates more.

Another hypothesis submits that calorically dense delectables over-stimulate reward centers in the brain, which escalates a desire for more food.

Many researchers feel personality traits can run in families. Placid versus active personalities show up even in infants, and weight differences vary according to activity levels.

Think back to high school. Look for a connection between your life events and your weight. What eating programs worked and which diets didn't?

Are you on any medications? Do you have any medical problems? Do you have a history of depression? Who else is in your home? What kind of support system do you have? What is your work atmosphere like?

Instead of saying, "I will eat less fat," propose a more specific initiative, "I will not spread butter on my toast on Tuesdays and Thursdays."

Find your triggers that cause you to eat inappropriately. Intercede in the chain of events before a binge occurs.

Food diaries are useful. They raise awareness of your eating. Your diary helps you uncover unconscious sabotage—like the bag of fat-free potato chips you scarfed down during the Cowboys game.

Losing weight is easy, keeping it off is the hard part. Figure out situations that caused you to binge.

Less than perfect eating is not a reason to give up. Just get back on track for your next meal. There is no such thing as a forbidden food. No one eats perfectly. Give yourself a break.

Other Influences. Sociologist have found that weight goes with the economy. When times are good, "thin is in," when there is economic depression, "plumper is better."

Because our culture values leanness, there is a lot of dieting, leading to diet induced obesity.

Restricting carbohydrates can lead to muscle loss, kidney problems, and acidosis. Low carbohydrate fad diets are popular every few years, but what you end up losing is water and muscle.

Redux and Phen-Fen are now off the market due to heart valve problems. Orlistat binds with about thirty percent of dietary fat and is excreted. Dexatrim (Phenylpropanolamine) decreases appetite for a week to ten days before the body adapts and it no longer has an effect. It has the potential to cause rapid heart beat and palpitations. People abused it because they assumed if a little was good, more was better. Amphetamines raise the metabolism. They were used extensively in the 1960's. Some doctors continue to prescribe them.

Ergogenic Aids. An ergogenic aid is a substance that is supposed to enhance martial arts performance. About 204 million dollars are spent each year by athletes trying to gain a millisecond edge over their opponents.

In interviews with 290 Olympic hopefuls, athletes were asked if they would take an untested drug to gain an advantage. Ninety-five percent said they would. The follow-up question inquired whether they would take the drug even if they knew it would cause them harm in the future. Ninety percent of those athletes answered "yes."

Belief in ergogenic aids has been around since there has been competition. In ancient Greece, athletes concluded eating powdered lion's teeth increased strength. In the early 1900's athletes assumed that extra protein provided additional power.

Athletes are always looking for a secret formula to boost performance. Some enjoy the placebo effect. That is, they believe a pill will help them improve, so it does. This psychological benefit is okay, unless serious money is wasted or there are unwanted side effects.

Creatine phosphate (CP) is considered a magic bullet in the bodybuilding/athletic world, even by today's standards. It provides a small reserve of quick energy during your workouts. The energy released from the breakdown of Adenosine Tri-Phosphate ATP and CP sustain all out, short duration, exercise such as during weight training.

Creatine is an amino acid. It is stored in your muscles as phosphocreatine. Horror stories of harmful side effects are unsubstantiated. Unpublished side effects, which have not been proven, include kidney failure, muscle cramps, strains, and pulls.

During intense activity, phosphocreatine is broken down into creatine and phosphate. This releases energy that regenerates ADP into ATP. ATP is the energy your muscles use to lift weights, punch, or kick.

About one-half pound of raw meat contains only a single gram of creatine. And you receive about half of your creatine from animal protein. The other half is made by your body. But when you use creatine supplementation, your body stops manufacturing its own creatine.

Research studies have shown that you can use creatine supplements to increase the storage of creatine in your muscles by about forty percent. In addition to creatine's ability to energize your ATP to be used for your training, there is a voluminizing effect to your muscles. That is, your body holds onto water and stores it in your muscles, making your muscles appear larger. It is unclear whether creatine actually stimulates protein synthesis to increase your muscle fiber size.

Controversy exists whether martial artists should do a loading phase of twenty grams of creatine daily for a week, prior to a maintenance phase. The maintenance dose is 2 to 5 grams of creatine per day. Megadoses of creatine create expensive urine and is not linked to greater muscle gains. But there is some evidence that taking glucose along with creatine increases the amount of creatine your muscles are able to store.

A variety of investigations have demonstrated that creatine does improve performance in high intensity, repetitive exercises like weight training and sprinting. There is no evidence however, that creatine improves a single bout of exercise, or long distance, endurance events.

If you are doing outdoor martial arts training in extreme heat, be careful not to use creatine. Its dehydrating effects are a concern.

Oxygen tanks are seen on the sidelines of professional football and basketball teams. Studies indicate however, that there is no known performance benefit to supplementing more "pure" oxygen than your body needs.

Carbohydrates provide energy to your muscles for both short and long distance activities. Products such as Gatorlode provide 140 grams of carbohydrate and Carboplex provides 164 grams. PowerBars and TigerSport Bars contain in excess of forty carbohydrate grams per bar. Carbohydrates consumed both before and after exercise helps you maintain a full load of muscle glycogen to power your workouts.

Vitamins are important to martial arts performance but the jury is out concerning the benefits of vitamin supplementation. Try to get most of your vitamins from fruits, vegetables, whole grain cereals, meat, and poultry. The proper combination of minerals are important to regulatory functions of the body.

Important Vitamins

- Vitamin C enhances immunity and is an antioxidant (antioxidants combat free radicals that "rust" your organs).
- Thiamine helps maintain your central nervous system.
- Niacin aids energy production and synthesis of fat and amino acids.
- Pyridoxine helps protein metabolism.
- Folacin aids new cell growth and red blood cell production.
- Vitamin E is an antioxidant.

High doses of vitamins and improper balance of minerals may be toxic to your body. For example, too much vitamin A can cause neurological problems, while an excess of one mineral can interfere with the function of another. Of the many known nutrients, only protein, carbohydrates, fats, vitamins A and C, thiamin, niacin, and calcium, are deemed necessary for high level functioning.

Caffeine in small dosages enhances endurance performance in elite and recreational martial artists. One theory is that caffeine spares glycogen in muscle and utilizes free fatty acids for energy. In addition, caffeine increases alertness and decreases fatigue. Finally, caffeine may improve sodium, potassium, and calcium balance within the working muscles.

Although caffeine has no nutritional value, and is often abused, caffeinated drinks consumed moderately, pose no health threats. Moderation has been defined as two cups of coffee or five glasses of iced tea a day.

Surveys show coffee drinkers smoke more often, get less exercise, and eat fattier meats. Tea drinkers seem to exercise more and eat better quality foods.

Previously, it was thought that coffee increased chances for breast cancer and fibrocystic breast disease. Recent research however, suggests none of this. Problems may develop however, if you drink coffee, cokes, and tea instead of beneficial beverages such as water and non-fat milk.

If you are anemic, and you must drink coffee, ingest your coffee before your meals. Polyphenols in caffeinated beverages interfere with iron absorption.

Addiction to caffeine is rampant. Stimulating your adrenals with a quick coffee fix is habit forming. You know you are hooked if you feel drowsy, fatigued, or experience headaches when you go cold turkey.

Caffeine mobilizes free fatty acids from your blood stream. This spares glycogen in your muscles. This means you may be able to train in your martial art a little longer and harder.

Ironically if you are a frequent caffeine user, there is less martial arts benefit. Therefore, if your goal is to drink caffeine to improve your martial arts performance, use it strategically, not constantly.

Important Minerals

- Calcium aids in bone formation, enzyme reactions, and muscle contractions.
- Magnesium is required for energy production, muscle relaxation, and nerve conduction.
- Sodium is responsible for nerve impulses, muscle action, and maintaining body fluid balances.
- Zinc helps with tissue growth, healing and immunity.
- Selenium is an antioxidant.

Experiment with caffeine in your training long before you use it during a tournament. Caffeine makes some people nervous and can cause stomach upset. And because caffeine is a diuretic, be sure to locate the nearest restroom.

Carnitine is alleged to metabolize fat so you lose weight. In reality, carnitine facilitates the transfer of fatty acids into the mitochondria where they are burned for fuel. There is no evidence however that carnitine decreases body fat.

Choline was purported to increase strength and decrease body fat. This product has not been shown to facilitate either of these claims.

Chromium is a trace mineral found in mushrooms, prunes, cereals, whole grain breads, and nuts. It is not readily absorbed in the body, so supplement manufacturers bound chromium with picolinate to ease absorption into the system.

Chromium picolinate was introduced to the American public in the 1980's. Early research suggested one 200 microgram tablet taken daily could help you gain muscle and lose fat. Imprecise measurement techniques in those studies were discovered, and the research was deemed faulty. When experimenters tried to replicate their results, there was no significant gain in muscle or decrease in body fat.

Furthermore, recent anecdotal reports suggest that excess chromium picolinate may cause anemia, chromosome damage, and cognitive impairment. (One 200 microgram tablet of chromium each day costs about forty-three cents.)

Coenzyme Q 10 has been used as a supplement for years in Japan as an aid to endurance. Studies have shown no benefit.

> ### Caffeine Content of Coffee, Tea, Soft Drinks, and Pain Relievers:
>
> - 10 ounces of instant coffee—130 mg.
> - 12 ounces of iced tea—70 mg.
> - 12 ounces of Coke—30 mg.
> - 12 ounces of Diet Coke—41 mg.
> - 12 ounces of Mountain Dew—55 mg.
> - 2 tablets of Anacin—64 mg.
> - 2 tablets of Excedrin—130 mg.

Ginseng is a wonder drug from Asia that is supposed to be a cure-all. There has not been enough research to demonstrate any benefits however.

Lecithin is an emulsifying agent and helps in digestion and absorption of fat. The body produces ample amounts of lecithin, therefore supplementation will not decrease body fat as suggested.

Metabolic bars such as PR Bars are comprised of forty percent carbohydrate, thirty percent protein, and thirty percent fat. They have not been shown to increase fat metabolism as suggested in the advertisements.

Protein. Protein needs range from 0.8 grams per kilogram of body weight to 2.0 grams of protein per kilogram of body weight. Heavy cardiovascular and strength training requires additional protein. Peter Lemon, Ph.D. recommends high-level athletes consume a gram of protein per pound of body weight. For most people, there is no need for supplementation.

Melatonin. Melatonin is advertised to promote sleep, alleviate jet-lag, combat aging, reduce the risk of cancer and heart disease, boost your immune system, improve your sex life, and lower your blood pressure and cholesterol.

Melatonin is a hormone produced by the pineal gland in the brain in response to darkness. Production decreases with age. It's function is to promote sleep.

Melatonin assists in the cycle of waking and sleeping. Production begins when a signal from the eye indicates darkness. It peaks at 2:00 A.M. and subsides by morning.

Melatonin may also act as an antioxidant. It is present in meats fruits, vegetables, and grains.

Children and adolescents produce an abundance of Melatonin. Production declines at puberty and continues to decrease through adulthood.

There appears to be minimal side effects when three milligrams of Melatonin are taken as a sleep aid. Some people report nightmares. It is contraindicated for folks on tranquilizers, anti-depressants, or sedatives, however. And high dosages may prevent ovulation.

Melatonin is a hormone. Recommendations from the scientific community suggest to wait for more studies before using it.

Sugar-free products are often used to wash down a candy bar. Maybe martial artists are thinking a diet soft drink has ten teaspoons less sugar than a regular one, and that they are saving calories. Or possibly they wouldn't have eaten the candy bar if they had chosen a sugared drink in the first place. Or perhaps the candy bar was a reward for stomaching a sugarless drink.

Regardless of the motivation, there seems to be at least two good reasons to use artificial sweeteners. The first is to prevent tooth decay. The second is to add some flavor to an otherwise sugar-less diabetic diet.

However there is no evidence that sugar-free products help people reduce calories or prevent obesity. The same with fat-free products. Some people think fat-free means calorie-free, so they gulp a whole box of fat-free cookies in a single sitting.

Taking in less saturated fat is beneficial from the standpoint of dropping total blood cholesterol. But it is also true that to lose weight you must create a calorie deficit by burning up more calories than you consume.

Using sugar and fat-free products may help you cut down, but you cannot trick your body into "thinking" it is taking in less calories. And because dosages of aspartame have not been proven safe, you should only ingest these products in moderation.

Amino acids are the building blocks of protein. Bodybuilders and martial artists have been popping these for years. The RDA suggests we only need 0.8 grams of protein per kilogram of bodyweight each day. However recent research by Lemon and Gontzen demonstrated that endurance athletes and weight trainers need between 1.2 and 1.8 grams of protein per kilogram of lean mass each day. They hypothesized that increased amino acids promoted protein synthesis and decreased muscle loss during heavy strength and endurance training. (Generic amino acids cost about two dollars per day.)

DHEA (Dehydroepiandrosterone) is touted as the fountain of youth. It is advertised to increase muscle, decrease body fat, and increase energy. DHEA is produced in the adrenal gland and is an androgen. It is found in yams and sold in health food stores.

Only a few carefully performed studies have been performed on DHEA. Two investigations reported significant increases in androgenic steroid blood levels along with feelings of physical and psychological well being. It is still unknown whether DHEA actually increases muscle and reduces fat.

Side effects include hair loss, voice deepening, and irreversible virilization in women. Without longitudinal studies it is difficult to predict long term effects. One group of researchers suggest that if DHEA truly increases circulating testosterone, then it may predispose men to prostate cancer. (DHEA costs about $1.30 per day.)

HMB (beta hydroxy beta methylbutyrate) is a metabolite of the branched chain amino acid leucine. You can find HMB naturally occurring in breast milk, catfish, and citrus fruit. HMB is purported to decrease protein catabolism (breakdown) so you can actually increase your muscle mass. Research in animals and humans have been favorable. Studies demonstrated that human subjects taking between 1.5 to 3.0 grams of HMB daily, showed significant gains in muscle. No side effects from taking HMB have been seen, but further research is needed. (HMB costs about $2.50 per day.)

Alternative Therapies. Lots of martial artists are turning to alternative approaches to curing their ailments. Especially when conventional methods fail. Magnet therapy, acupuncture, chiropractic, and meditation are some of the techniques that are gaining in popularity. Back pain sufferers, who have tried everything else, are ready to give anything a chance.

Before you pay good money for an alternative healing technique, do your homework. Interview your prospective healer/guru just as you would your medical doctor. If your healer requires you to undergo expensive testing, followed by the promise of a miracle cure, run the other way.

Check on your therapist's credentials. Is he/she certified? Phone their national certifying organization with specific questions.

Acupuncture is a Chinese art of healing. Thin needles are placed in strategic body parts to redirect energy flow. Skeptics theorize the needles act as a counter-irritant, similar to heat balm. The National Institute of Health (NIH) recently suggested that acupuncture may be useful as an adjunct modality. Recent studies have shown that acupuncture, combined with conservative therapies, may be helpful in treating carpal tunnel syndrome, low back pain, fibromyalgia, and tennis elbow.

Chiropractors use spinal manipulation along with exercise, physical therapy, and rehab procedures to help their patients. Chiropractic techniques have been found especially useful in treating acute lower back pain in adults.

Hyperbaric oxygen is in vogue. You may have noticed professional athletes on the sidelines sucking extra oxygen in an attempt to improve their performance. There is no evidence to date however, suggesting more oxygen actually helps athletes play better. In fact, although hyperbaric chambers have been used to speed healing in crush injuries, compartment syndromes, and decompression sickness, there seems to be no hyperbaric benefit to muscle injuries, ligament tears, and sprains.

Magnet therapy is a multi-level marketing program. People swear by the healing power of magnets. Some place them strategically under mattresses, or embedded into the soles of their shoes. These unpaid or paid testimonials declare that magnets cured their aches and pains. Benjamin Franklin did an early investigation on the benefits of magnet therapy. He painted blocks of wood black, and told patients they were magnets. Sure enough, painted wood healed those who believed. There has been a dearth of empirical research on magnets however, except for a few studies with very small sample sizes. Current research suggests that magnets may be best applied by helping to unite bone fractures.

Massage therapy has been around for centuries. There is little argument that massage feels good. And there are a variety of different types of massage therapies. From long, gliding, surface, techniques to deep tissue pummeling, to sports massage. Recent research verifies that massage reduces muscle soreness after exercise. And some athletes are using massage as a tool to prevent injury.

Relaxation techniques have been shown to reduce stress. Some medical practitioners use relaxation strategies to successfully treat their chronic pain patients. These relaxation techniques include:

- Imagining yourself in a peaceful scene.
- Progressively contracting and relaxing all of your muscles until you are very relaxed.
- Deep breathing, and meditation.
- Many studies have demonstrated the stress-busting effects of these mind/body applications.

Tai Chi is a Chinese martial art performed in extreme slow motion, supported by deep, relaxed breathing and a concentrated mind. Empirical studies have demonstrated that Tai Chi can help older adults improve their balance, strength, flexibility, and endurance. Tai Chi also helps to reduce tension, stress, and anxiety. And because Tai Chi is low impact, there is little stress on the joints.

Martial Arts Mindset: Injury and Rehabilitation. Many who are not injured do not workout in the martial arts. Others, such as yourself, cannot train in your martial art because of an injury. Healthy individuals who do not workout are the same as those who are injured and cannot workout. But those of you who are injured and rehabilitate, can continue your workouts. You are the role models for your sedentary counterparts.

Martial artists are relaxed, confident, and focused. That is, until they are injured. Imagine that your livelihood depended on your fitness, or health. In the heat of sparring, you hear a loud pop and are crippled with pain. Lactic acid is one thing, but the debilitating pain that sidelines you is physically and mentally crushing.

CHAPTER FOUR

Injuries

An injury can be disheartening. Physical pain is only part of it. Impairments can decrease confidence and increase fear. You may wonder if you will ever be the same. The pain may be so severe that you do not think you can handle another day.

In the dojo, martial artists are in control. They are experts at handling their emotions. Fighting an opponent is easy compared to battling an injury.

At the onset of an acute injury, many martial artists are basket cases. "Why me?" they say. Their injury dictates their level of thinking. They ride an emotional roller coaster, at first feeling sorry for themselves, and sometimes leading to a mild or serious form of clinical depression. Fortunately, support from family, friends, senseis, and dojo mates may get them through the crisis phase. Once reality has set in, martial artists must deal with the problems at hand and begin planning.

But martial artists are looking for specific answers. "How badly am I injured?" "How long will my injury last?" "Can I return to my martial arts next week or next year?" "What are my options?" "Can I use rehab to get me through?" "Or is there a need for emergency surgery?" These questions usually revolve around the nature of the injury and the diagnosis involved.

The medical clinic the martial artists select must understand their situation and know how to react to different personalities and realities. The medical team needs to bring understanding and meaning to the physical, mental, emotional, and spiritual aspect of healing.

Rehabilitation

After martial artists see their physicians, regardless if it is non-operative or there will be surgical intervention, they will generally see a rehabilitation specialist. It is here that clinicians teach martial artists to use their tenacious, win-at-all-cost spirit to speed their recovery. Just as a shaman understands his patients belief system before prescribing a cure, rehab specialists probe their athletes mind/spirit, not just their injuries. The rehab clinicians help patient/martial artists set short and long term recovery goals. Their mission is to turn their patients "will-to-win" into a "will-to-recover."

The "rehabilitation of the mind" is one of the key factors in recovery. Martial artists can sense this one-on-one approach. And because of the varying personalities encountered, this approach is task specific for all martial artists. Martial artists are sent with a checklist of activities that the physician has requested. The injury will dictate the activity list, but it can be as simple as range of motion exercises, or it may require a clinician sitting down with each patient and describing a more extensive program. If there are certain modalities the physician requests, patients will begin this program immediately along with any range of motion exercise. Again, the protocol will vary according to the diagnosis, and whether the injury was acute or chronic.

Some martial artists become over-zealous, however. They think that if a few repetitions are good, a lot are better. Overtraining during recovery leads to meltdown. That's why there is constant communication between patients and their rehab specialists. Long after patients are released the dialogue continues. One of the best customer services a rehabilitation clinic can establish is telephone contact with their patients.

Recovery is not just physical. Recuperation is emotional. Look on the bright side to being sidelined. You probably needed the rest. Or maybe overtraining caused your injury in the first place. Take a break. Enjoy your time off. See yourself from the inside-out. In the heat of battle, day after day, year after year it is difficult to be objective. Use your down time to assess your strengths and liabilities. Time off provides you the opportunity to balance your priorities. It is easy to get caught up. Let your convalescence heal your outer and inner self.

If a martial artist injures her right knee, twenty-five percent of the body has some down or mild activity time. The other seventy-five percent can be working towards improvement. Rehab specialists usually suggest workouts for maintenance with the left leg since initially the left will take the brunt of an acute and sometimes chronic injury. In fact, if there are certain flaws or weaknesses to be worked on; rehab specialists prescribe it during their rehabilitation program. Martial artists should return stronger than prior to the injury. This concerted effort and focus on rehabilitation really allows martial artists extreme concentration, not only physically, but also mentally. In fact rehab specialists council martial artists to utilize time away from their art to develop outer and inner strength. Rather than brooding, martial artists use techniques such as mental imagery to speed their healing.

Close your eyes and relax. Imagine yourself performing your sport. See it, feel it, experience it. You are strong, fast, and agile. Better than you have ever been before. Now take a few moments to use that same energy to focus on your rehab. See your range of motion improving. Feel your muscles growing stronger. Experience healing.

Rest is recovery. Under-resting is overtraining. Take an inventory of your body. What needs work? Increase your upper body strength if your legs require rehabilitation. A weight lifters, muscles are torn down in the gym. Their muscles grow with rest. You may surprise yourself and return to your training with a better attitude. It is like starting over. Everything is fresh and new.

When you are finally ready to return to training, be sure you receive medical clearance. There should be no doubt about your wellness. Do not risk a relapse. Sleep well, eat correctly, and train moderately. You should be comfortable about your workouts.

Mind & Body

Hippocrates said that a patient should be at the helm of his own healing. Herbert Benson, Harvard cardiologist went on to say, "Ideally, medicine should be a three-legged stool, with the legs of surgery and pharmaceuticals balanced with spiritual self-care, such as meditation or prayer. But often this third leg is missing."

Benson asserts that sixty to ninety percent of all illness is brought on by stress. Surgery and pharmaceuticals do little to curtail stress.

Martial arts meditation, "reciting a prayer, focusing on a particular image, word or physical motion (like the heel-to-toe rocking that Orthodox Jews do during worship) is a balm for an amazing number of ailments" according to Dr. Benson.

Stress-related disorders are benefited by spiritual practice. During meditation and prayer, breathing is long and deep, and the heart beats slower.

Breathing is useful, but faith is associated with increased health and longevity. There have been more than three hundred studies on the effects of faith on healing. Seventy five percent of those have shown that believing in a higher power is good for your health. Deeply religious people exhibit a longer life expectancy, quicker recovery, better quality of life, lower rates of depression and substance abuse. Every culture has a belief in some sort of higher power. Belief is empowering.

A study at Dartmouth College revealed the best predictor of heart bypass survival rates was whether patients believed in God. Six months after surgery, twelve percent of non-believers died. One hundred percent of believers were still living.

A 1996 study at Salem College showed that spiritual practice had a more significant effect on blood pressure than whether the patients smoked, drank, or ate a high fat/calorie diet.

Martial artists are physically, socially, and mentally stimulated almost all of the time. It is increasingly difficult to find time to be alone. Lunch hour has turned into catch-up. Midmorning breaks are nonexistent. Cellular phones, megachurches, pagers, and fax machines are a bane to quiet time.

Information provides tools to improve your life. Martial arts instructors spur you on. Networking enhances your communication. Martial arts training makes you better. But you need privacy to figure it all out. Give yourself a few moments to gain perspective.

After an hour in a sensory deprivation tank, subjects experienced lower blood pressure, improved creativity, a more positive outlook, and higher mental functioning. Solitude allows you to get organized.

Creative youngsters cherish their time alone. My eight-year-old boy spends several hours a week interacting with imaginary characters. At first, I thought this was peculiar. Now I understand that personal moments are a vital ingredient to enhanced creativity.

Being alone doesn't mean you are lonely. Eating lunch in the corner of a crowded cafeteria can be demoralizing. But it does not have to be. It depends on your attitude. Imagine yourself performing kata or sparring, or be mindful of your meal.

Some people think you are antisocial if you are unaccompanied. But martial arts is a socially acceptable methods of isolation. Close the door to your office and perform Tai Chi. In Japan there are places set aside specifically for people to unwind.

Some martial artists ultimately "say no" to crowded offices and harried lifestyles. For sanity's sake, they give up lucrative careers to pursue self-employment, or a more relaxed profession.

Discussions with friends and co-workers is helpful. And so are television and computer games. But a few moments of quiet contemplation can do wonders. Martial arts masters focus their chi. Zen masters contemplate koans. Thoreau circumambulated Walden Pond.

Use solitary moments to provide insight. Deepak Chopra stated, "you are those moments between your thoughts." Value personal time to discover who you are. Become sensitive to your thoughts, actions, and behaviors.

After a hard day, when you open your front door, ask for ten minutes. Relax. Prioritize. Flip on your answering machine. What phone call could be more important than finding sanity? Pamper yourself. Listen to music and practice a kata. Detachment is an end in itself.

Beyond Pain

Nerves send lactic acid pain messages to the spinal cord, which delivers them to the brain. Sean McCann, sport psychologist at the Olympic Training Center, teaches athletes to use key words and imagery to reinterpret pain signals more positively. Pain diminishes when you call it something else. O. Carl Simonton, M.D., says to picture your lactic acid pain as a glowing orange ball. Then see your body fending off the pain (for example the lactic acid glowing orange ball disappearing).

An elite martial artist may describe discomfort as enjoyable, but another will never truly understand the description. McCann suggests "Don't say the pain of martial arts training will be over soon." You're surrendering. Learn and practice the art of association. Focus exclusively on your punches or kicks. You must be in control of your pain.

Place your palms five inches from each other. Imagine energy flowing from one palm to the other and back. Similarly, you can send blood to your legs to power your roundhouse kicks.

Disassociate from the boredom of jumping rope by picturing yourself in a peaceful scene. Imagine yourself tap-dancing on a cloud. Dissociation is setting the mind apart from the body. Plenty of world-class martial artists dissociate from the regularity and pain of their training. You can exercise through a multitude of drills in a seemingly few minutes if you dissociate by focusing on music.

Mental Toughness Tips

1. Stay pumped up even when you are tired or discouraged.
2. Act "as if" you are kicking well even when you are not.
3. Plan your strategy prior to each workout.

Or you can associate by recruiting every fiber of your hamstrings to pull through on your leg down or your ax kick. Changing your mind about discomfort can change your body.

Quitting is usually the first option when confronted with the fatigue and discomfort of martial arts training. But if your goal is to improve your martial arts skill, sometimes it is useful to persevere.

Expect to get through discomfort. Teach your body to handle discomfort a little at a time. Reach deep inside and ask a little more of yourself for each martial arts training session. The following two phases are designed to help you get through the pain:

Phase I
- Fatigue exists in your mind.
- You can beat fatigue and discomfort.
- Go with it. Pushing yourself through discomfort will lead you to your goal.
- Increase your kicking speed. Expect an increase in discomfort.
- An increase in "the burn" is a signal you are nearing the completion of your training.
- You are objective about the burn and fatigue. Observe it. Enjoy it.

Phase II
- You have the power to control your thoughts.
- Your mind can focus on only one thing at a time.
- When the lactic acid burn and fatigue become unbearable, change your focus.
- Become part of your surroundings.
- Dissociate, the discomfort will disappear.

Choose to associate with your body by "feeling" every aspect of your kicks. Visualize fibers splitting and blood pumping to your quadriceps, hamstrings, gluteals, gastrocnemius, and soleus.

While associating with your muscles, you will find random thoughts will enter your mind in the form of self-talk. Talk to yourself nicely. Self-talk takes the form of positive affirmations such as "Practicing my kicks will make me a better martial artist." These self-verbalizations raise arousal levels.

Although your arousal level may increase, relax your muscles. With relaxation comes speed and efficiency. Relax and notice if upper body muscles are wasting precious energy.

A simple way to increase your relaxation and speed is to use mental imagery. Picture yourself performing a perfect roundhouse kick. Several studies suggest that when a subject visualizes himself training, nervous impulses are sent down the proper neuromuscular pathways to stimulate muscle fibers enhancing speed and performance.

Breathing. Martial arts breathing is a natural stress-buster. Breathing is simple. You do it all day and night. You may not notice you inhale and exhale at least fifteen thousand times each day. But run after a bus, or swim the length of a pool under water. Then you realize how breathing, or the lack thereof, can affect every cell in your body.

Shallow, rapid breathing can trigger the fight or flight response. Breathe like a Zen monk and you will relax.

Practice your breathing anywhere, anytime. Breathe naturally and deeply from your diaphragm. Instead of squeezing your tummy within the confines of a tightly notched belt, relax a little and belly breathe from your abdomen. Your lungs take in more oxygen.

A variety of breathing gurus teach different skills and drills. One strategy teaches you to breathe in through one nostril and out the other. Another instructs you to focus on the temperature and vibration of the air as it passes through your nasal passages. Breathing is a first step in your mind/body connection.

When you are anxious, your body prepares for a crisis. Blood is quickly transported to your muscles for fight or flight. Your blood pressure increases and so does your heart rate. And to exhale carbon dioxide more quickly, you breathe faster.

To get the oxygen you need, without thinking, you breathe erratically from your chest. Exhaling carbon dioxide too quickly disturbs your blood pH. This keeps your blood from efficiently getting oxygen to your brain, muscles, and organs. Some estimates suggest that sixty to ninety percent of medical ailments are stress related.

When you inhale-exhale impulsively, you hyperventilate. And if you are anxious all day long, you may be in a constant state of hyperventilation. You may be hyperventilating at this very moment.

The lower lobes of your lungs lie below your chest. Breathe deeply and allow air to fill this area. This is diaphragmatic breathing.

Muscle tension, especially tight abdominals, constrict your diaphragm. So does holding your stomach in to appear svelte. Wearing a tight belt teaches you to breathe improperly too.

Take a deep breath from your belly. This short circuits your sympathetic nervous system and lessens your stress reaction. Automatically your heart rate and blood pressure drop.

Focus on your breathing. Simply take your mind off of the distressing situation. Breathing occupies your thoughts. Just by altering your attention, you decrease your anxiety. There is no room for negativity. Pain patients use breathing techniques to lessen their discomfort and increase relaxation.

Your lower lungs inflate with less effort than your upper lungs. But you probably do not take advantage of this. Count your inhalations. You probably inhale about twenty times per minute.

Try taking in more air with each breath. Fill your lungs. This allows you to breathe slower. Breathing smoothly helps stabilize your blood pH. Belly breathers average eight to fourteen inhalations per minute.

Your thoughts can provoke anxiety. Anxiety may lead to stress. Breath observation will help you calm down. Breathe in through your nose by inhaling for a count of ten. Hold for five seconds and release your breath through your mouth for a count of five. Relax all of the muscles in your body. Focus only on your breathing. Follow your breath. Allow your mind to drift. Breathing is a very powerful relaxation technique.

CHAPTER 5

Minding Fitness

Focus

Researchers at the Dallas Aerobic Center have demonstrated stress reduction and longevity benefits when exercising in a relaxed cadence for twenty minutes.

Researchers have shown that when students are relaxed and focused they exhibit alpha brain waves. Alpha is propitious for learning and retaining information. Recent investigations determined that subjects analyzed and recalled more effectively while listening to music at sixty beats per minute, approximating the pattern of the human heart. Proponents of this instructional system maintain that if pupils review their lessons while attending to classical music they comprehend faster and assimilate more. Just as an infant snuggles close to hear her mother's heartbeat you can study along with your favorite tunes played at sixty beats per minute.

Most of us choose activities to escape. We prefer to watch sitcoms rather than listen to our thoughts. It's easier to read the newspaper than to do Tai Chi. Some combine reading the newspaper with family, dinner, and television. Our lives are about distractions. Just sitting is not easy.

Furthermore, we need diversions while we perform our activities. Weight lifters listen to blaring music and cyclists wear headphones. Listening to our bodies has become a lost art. It seems more efficient to "read" a book-on-tape than to attend to your breathing. It's easier to pump out that last repetition to Metallica than to focus on the muscle you are working.

Some folks tap their fingers and fidget to ease tension. Others meditate. Herbert Benson, a Harvard trained cardiologist has extolled the advantages of repeating a mono-syllabic phrase to reduce stress and improve well-being. His studies with transcendental meditators demonstrated that a few minutes of quiet repetition can manifest tremendous physiological gains.

I was a teenager when I first enrolled in a meditation class. The teacher taught us to recite a mantra, a word theoretically designed for each of us. We were instructed to repeat this mantra (mine was "ing") silently for twenty minutes. If distracting thoughts or sounds disturbed us we were advised to allow them proceed through one ear and out the other. When we thought twenty minutes was up, we were to open one eye and glance at a timepiece. Occasionally I awakened from a deep sleep with my chin nestled on my chest.

Deep rhythmic breathing is another centering strategy. Breathe from your diaphragm instead of your chest. To accomplish this, lie on your back. Place your left hand on your chest and your right hand on your stomach. Inhale from your nose taking five seconds to expand your lungs. Focus on lowering your diaphragm. Let the air fill your lower, central, and upper chest, in that order. Then take seven seconds to exhale through your mouth by raising your diaphragm. Only your right hand should move as you breathe deeply from your abdomen.

To combine meditation with deep breathing sit erect and take a deep breath from your diaphragm, then exhale. Relax. Focus on your breath. Let nothing distract or disturb you; just breathe. If thoughts or sounds interfere, notice them but let them go. Close this book, close your eyes, and continue. After five minutes, slowly come out of your relaxed state. How do you feel? Close your eyes and continue relaxing for twenty minutes. Caution—do not lie down unless your goal is sleep.

Mind/Body Psyche

Martial artists sometimes neglect the cognitive phase of their workouts. They spend hours physically preparing and they know the mental aspect of their performance is important, but they spend little time in mental preparation.

Getting psyched is extremely important to exemplary achievement. Knowing when to turn it on will help you be your best. Mike Tyson throws punches with "malicious intent." World Karate Champion, Bill Wallace pummels opponents with vicious left foot attacks. These champions summon all of their physical and mental strength to win. But their emotions hardly enter the ring. Punching and kicking is their craft. They are workmanlike in their devastation.

Preparing for a martial arts tournament requires a tremendous amount of mental readiness. During idle moments your attention shifts to your upcoming contest. Your mind prepares your body for battle. Stomachs rumble, muscles tighten, and palms sweat. This "fight or flight response" is distressing to some. "Would be" competitors cannot handle tension. Their bodies become ill. Or they stumble and sprain ankles. Their sparring buddies say, "tough luck." They were simply not prepared to compete.

More likely, they may have been physically ready but not mentally fit. It is easy to exaggerate the caliber of adversaries or the magnitude of an event. Rather than viewing competition as win-lose, success-fail; approach each match as instruction. In a single tournament you will learn more about yourself than in six months of training. Competition brings out your best. Spectators increase your arousal amplifying the urgency of your event. The better prepared you are, the more an audience will spur you on. For a few moments you are on the edge. It is electrifying. You may transcend your limits. Give yourself an opportunity to be your best.

Emotions are a double edged sword. They increase your intensity but multiply your chances for error. Counterproductive feelings sabotage your performance. Defensiveness and negative emotions weaken you. Rage tears your game plan apart. During intense competition you may feel frustrated and experience antagonism. In anticipation of a tantrum, plan a response. Set limits on your emotional behavior. Promise yourself not to succumb. No matter how bad things become, acknowledge your opponent for issuing a challenge. The tougher he is, the more you will mature.

You have no control over your opponent's techniques or his personality, so focus on your performance. If your rival displays malevolence, ignore him. When your opponent rages, use his misplaced energy to fuel your tenacity and courage. Develop a system. Emotions take a back seat. You cannot be enraged and centered at the same time.

In a tournament you may compete for only a few minutes. The remainder of your time is spent waiting. Structure this respite to prepare for your subsequent bout. Begin thinking about your next opponent immediately. Don't exalt yourself until the tournament is over. Consider the plight of the defending heavyweight World Taekwondo Champion from Germany, Dirk Jung. He beat me in the finals of the Asian Games in Taiwan just two months earlier. He was primed to win a second straight World Championship in front of his home crowd in Stuttgart, Germany. The round before we fought, he had a ferocious fray with the Korean. Jung celebrated his conquest with a victory lap. He rejoiced and probably felt the battle was over. His body was in a recovery mode, leaving him too relaxed, flat. It was difficult for him to regroup and be his emotional best for our fight. He lost.

Do not permit a negative attitude to limit your performance. Hostility can affect your confidence and concentration. Transform fear or anger into focused energy. Start with relaxation. And than concentrate. Mental preparation is a skill. A disciplined mind does not come fast or easy. If you try too hard you may undermine your efforts. Ask yourself, "Why am I competing?" Think about the reasons you began.

Stress

You might assume most cardiovascular disease is correlated with high-fat eating, smoking, or sedentary living. A major predictor of heart disease is job dissatisfaction. Heart attacks are plentiful Monday mornings at 9:00 A.M.

Another predictor of heart disease is whether you think you are happy. Happiness is not just a few moments of exhilaration.

From the moment you were born you were bombarded with movements, sights, and sounds. Life provided you with stimuli. You learned how to perceive your environment. The physical world existed in direct response to your treatment of it. If you just won the World Martial Arts Championships vs. learning you had heart disease, your physiology would change dramatically.

In an experiment, mice in Group A were injected with a substance to increase their immune system. Mice in Group B were injected with the same substance, and were simultaneously exposed to the aroma of camphor. Subsequently after the mice in Group B inhaled camphor (without the injection), their immune cells were elevated.

This research is similar to the classical conditioning paradigm you may have studied in high school:

Dogs were presented with food—they salivated.
Dogs were offered food while a bell chimed—they salivated.
Dogs heard a bell chime—they salivated.

This is called a conditioned response. You are not a mouse or a dog, but you can be conditioned to react to a stimuli. Begin with your thinking. The average human has 60,000 thoughts per day. Brain cells communicate with the cells in your body. Immune cells have receptor sites that are constantly eavesdropping on your musings.

Thinking leads to a response. If you are negative, depressed, and despondent, your immune cells will weaken. Inadvertent habits may prompt you to repeat biochemical and behavioral processes that bring about illness (e.g. stress related disease).

You react according to your thoughts. Harness your thoughts and feelings to benefit yourself and others. A positive, winning attitude strengthens your immunity. At the Simonton Institute in Fort Worth, terminally ill patients were taught to attack their cancer at the cellular level. Children imagined white knights destroying evil cancer cells. In some cases there were remissions.

You are a bundle of conditioned reflexes, stimulated daily. Psycho neuro immunology (PNI) is a revolutionary science whose practitioners study the relationship between mind and body.

Be the benefactor instead of the victim of your thoughts. Use your thoughts, but don't allow them to use you. Place most of your attention on the positive. Be proactive.

Radiate hope and prepare yourself for excellent health. View yourself not just as a physical body, but as a place where optimism resides. Do not confuse the car and the driver. You are your thoughts.

Some of your thoughts are habit. If a novice student unwittingly kicks you in the groin, your initial response might be "what is wrong with this guy? I'll kill him." Short-circuit reactive thinking by changing your mindset. Remind yourself not to allow external circumstances to compel you to anger. You are the thinker of your thought. In the spaces between thoughts you are in control. Do not react to situations like everyone else.

Overtraining

Some martial artists maximize the value of every jump or stretch in order to justify the time expenditure—even if their purpose for training was stress management or peace of mind.

I received both truth and fiction from my early mentors. Before a professional full-contact fight my trainer rubbed Bengay all over me. I was on fire. I came out so hard and fast I had no punches or kicks left for the last round. Fortunately neither did my opponent.

Two weeks prior to the World Taekwondo Championships in Stuttgart, we trained on German time. We set our alarms for 2:00 A.M., trained all day and tried to sleep at 7:00 P.M.

Most of us were sleep deprived and miserable. We neglected to consider late flights or layovers. By the time we reached Germany it took several days for our overtrained bodies to recover from severe jet lag.

Most mammals are on a strict schedule of activity and recovery. Cats are notorious for lounging, but when it's time for action they pounce. Martial arts is high intensity too, requiring rest periods between bursts of activity. Rejuvenate yourself between bouts of exertion. Intense effort is followed by recovery, where you prepare for your next campaign. The goal is to maximize intensity and increase your capacity to handle it.

Set performance goals to determine training time and energy expenditure. But goal setting is a double edged sword. Effortless ambitions aren't worthy. And if your goal is too extravagant it becomes your personal nightmare. Daily training should be motivational and energetic. Be sure you are on track.

Enjoy a vibrant lifestyle. Attaining short term goals provides you confidence for the long haul. Eating correctly, sleeping enough, and incremental improvements in strength, flexibility, and endurance can be measured. These assessments should satisfy you day-to-day.

Pushing to the limit feels good. But maybe that is wrong. Contemporary martial artists follow season-long training schedules. They know exactly how much time to jump rope, lift weights, run, and stretch from January until December. And then they start all over again. They claim they need structure in their training to have an idea of what they can accomplish.

Elite martial artists realize the benefits of force pads and heart rate monitors to regulate their training. Anaerobic threshold, maximum heart rate, pressure indicators, and digitized biomechanical analysis, allow athletes to maximize their training time. More and more contemporary martial artists believe in scientific training.

A little technology can reveal signs of overtraining. Signs of overtraining include:
- Elevated heart rate. If your heart rate is higher than normal when you awaken, you may be overtraining.
- Negative attitude. Inadequate recovery from training may lead to listlessness.
- Weight loss. Overtraining can lead to muscle loss and weakness.
- Lack of recovery. After a martial arts training session, you may recover slowly if you are overtrained because your immune system is depressed.
- Loss of interest. Overtraining leads to boredom and lack of commitment in your martial art.
- Fatigue. Overtraining causes fatigue from even a mild martial art training session.
- Injury. Overtraining may cause overuse injuries and muscle pain.

There is a push-pull, yin-yang, give-and-take that assures balance in your martial arts training. Workouts are interspersed with bouts of relaxation. Sometimes you feel like doing a few extra katas. But if you do not eat enough, sleep well, or handle stress effectively, you overtrain.

Under-resting is over-training. Prevent over-training by scheduling rest periods and sleep. Restful activities may include reading, writing, television, eating, sleeping, and family time.

Martial arts training can have a positive effect on your immune system. Light workouts increase T-cells, which destroy viruses and cancer. The immune systems of one hundred men were monitored daily for eight months. Following pleasurable activities, immune function increased for two days.

But anything taken to extremes becomes detrimental, including martial arts. People who overtrain develop significantly more upper respiratory infections as compared to those who exercise in moderation.

If you become ill, listen to your body. Martial arts can be good for you, but heavy training triggers stress hormones that may interfere with your immune system's ability to fight virus or infection. If you have a virus with muscular aches and pains it is especially important to stay out of the studio until your symptoms disappear. Risk factors for colds and virus are:

- Eating fewer than three meals a day without fruits and vegetables.
- Exercising less than three days a week.
- Working with the general public.
- Working indoors in crowded conditions.
- Exposing yourself to friends, co-workers, and family who suffer with a cold.
- Get depressed easily.

Footwear, from the Ground Up

Know your foot. Learn the types of martial arts shoes available to you. Then you can make an informed purchase. Your foot has nineteen muscles, thirty-three joints, and twenty-six bones. It is an incredible creation.

Your feet are phenomenal. You land with six hundred pounds of force on each of several thousand footfalls, in just a few hours of martial arts.

Going barefoot while practicing works for some, but martial arts/cross-training shoes may provide support if you need it.

Purchasing sport shoes is an art. Allow a specially trained employee at an athletic shoe store to help you. But if you have very high arches, are flat-footed, or pronate, pay special attention to your style of shoe.

Your shoes should fit the contours of your feet to avoid heel spurs, hammer toes, plantar fasciitis, and a variety of other maladies caused by improper footwear. A minor alignment problem can wreak havoc in your feet, shins, knees, and lower back.

Narrow toe boxes may cause hammer toes, and other foot deformities. Tight shoes can produce bunions. Shoes that are too snug across the top-front of your foot may precipitate Morton's neuroma, a nerve problem.

For months I didn't realize that my tight martial arts shoes were intensifying pain. After suffering several analgesic injections, I wised-up and purchased a roomier shoe.

No two people have the same type of foot. Your foot may be high arched, flat, normal, or somewhere in between. A high arched foot does not absorb shock very well. It flexes poorly and under pronates so that when it strikes the ground it does not roll smoothly from heel to toe.

A flat foot overpronates which means that it rolls inward stressing the ankle and arch of the foot. A pronated foot leans inward with each step. The inside of the foot touches the ground first.

A normal foot lands on the outside of the heel and rolls easily onto the ball of the foot. It is the perfect shock absorber.

A high-arched foot under pronates (tilts outward) with each step. The outer side of the foot touches the ground first and the foot rolls inward. To combat supination, the form around a high-arched shoe is curved inward to encourage pronation. This fosters a heel-to-toe rocking chair motion that increases shock absorption. Some outsoles are gas or gel filled with a polyurethane midsole.

Flat feet have low or no arches. Low-arched feet require rigid support. The form around which the shoe is constructed should be straight or just slightly curved. Flat feet need torsion control shoes with anti-pronation devices. These include stiff heel counters, a firm midsole, and a solid outsole.

A normal foot performs well in a stable shoe with a semi-curved form. It requires a moderate blend of support and cushioning.

Find shoes that accommodate your feet. The average person needs a shoe that is not too soft, hard, or unstable.

Examine your shoes for wear. Set them on a table and inspect them from behind (Figure 5-1). If they slant toward each other you might be a pronator. If they tilt outward you may be a supinator with a high-arched foot. Your podiatrist can help you with this.

After a shower step onto a piece of cardboard. If the imprint of your foot is filled in so that most of the bottom of your foot is in contact with the ground, you may have flat feet. If there is a narrow band and considerable space between your forefoot and heel, you probably have high arches.

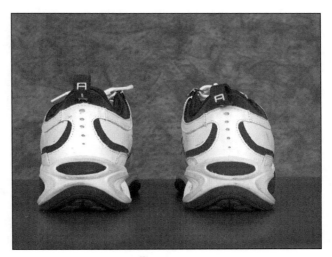

Figure 5-1

Be sure your shoes have cushion to support your weight. If you have high arches, you may need more cushioning. Arch pain may be alleviated with a simple arch support.

The inner sole includes a heel cup and arch support. It is the inside of your shoe. Your feet rest against the inner soles. You can replace the inner sole with orthotic devices made specifically for your foot.

Stabilizers should be built in to add control to brace your movements. Flat feet require stabilization to limit excess movement.

Years ago, midsoles were the limiting factor in your shoes. The midsole is a layer of cushion between the outer sole and inner sole. Their purpose is to absorb shock. They were fabricated from ethyl vinyl acetate or polyurethane foam. These materials didn't last very long.

Outer soles and the upper part of your shoes were smudge free. But after months of wear, midsoles secretly broke down. Midsoles flexed in the middle of your foot, creating impairments such as plantar fasciitis.

Now shoe manufacturers provide flexibility in the forefoot. Many top shoe companies provide air and gel midsoles. This high-tech design extends durability by fifty percent.

A new style of lacing termed "laceroni" has become popular. You may have seen these in hiking boots. This lacing system distributes pressure evenly across the top of your foot without kinking. The laces are rounded (ie. "roni") rather than flat. Rounded laces come untied more often than flat laces. But since laceroni is extra long, a double knot is an easy solution.

In years past, the top of shoes grated against your ankles, rubbing up and down with each step. Now the crowns of shoes are specially designed with neoprene sleeves. Instead of chafing, neoprene grips your ankles and provides a better fit.

Thinner midsoles are used for martial arts shoes to bring your feet closer to the floor. This provides a better "feel" without giving up padding. In addition, since your center of gravity is lowered, your balance is better, reducing your chance of ankle injury.

Don't forget about traction. If you slip on the floor you injure yourself. But if there is too much traction, as in a shoe that "sticks", you could blow out your knee on a roundhouse kick. Wear a shoe that affords a fair amount of friction, but will not cling to the floor.

Measure both of your feet properly to fit your shoes. Your feet swell as the day progresses, so purchase your shoes later in the day. And beware that your feet change size and shape as you age. Wear the same type of socks you use for your activity. New shoes do not have to be broken-in. They should feel good immediately.

Sleep

The quality of your sleep affects your martial arts workouts. And your workouts affect your sleep.

At the Olympic Training Center in Colorado Springs, Herb Perez, a member of the United States Taekwondo Team, was preparing for his debut in the Olympics. Herb confided he could not fall asleep the night before his matches. As a sport psychologist for the medical team, I suggested Herb not worry how well he sleep the night before his bout. What mattered was the quality of sleep the months-of-nights before his event. Herb went on to win a Gold Medal in the Olympic Games.

Forty million Americans have some sort of sleep problem. One in three have difficulty falling asleep. Americans today sleep an average of ninety minutes less than they did a century ago.

Alertness and visual skills may be impaired by minor sleep loss. But chronic sleep deprivation reduces your vigilance, mental abilities, muscle strength, and aerobic capacity.

Insomnia affects your ability to handle stress and solve problems. Lack of sleep can hinder your job performance. Not to mention the sleep-deprivation related disasters including Chernobyl and the Exxon Valdez. And how many accidents have you heard about where people have dozed at the wheel of their automobiles?

Maybe Jay Leno only needs three hours of sleep. And perhaps you need ten. A report in the *American Journal of Public Health* revealed that sleeping less than five hours, or more than ten hours increased mortality risk. The lowest death rates were reported in those who slept seven hours a night.

Sleeping aids and pills may be habit forming. Ironically, these products don't necessarily improve deep sleep. Similar to alcohol, they allow you to become drowsy, but some may actually impede quality sleep.

Martial arts training helps you fall asleep quicker and improve the quality of your deep sleep. Try working out during the day. Keep it moderate. Too much exercise, or training just before bedtime may be counterproductive. Late afternoon activity seems to be the best time to enhance your sleep.

> ## Try These Hints For Better Quality Sleep
>
> 1. Eat a snack before bedtime. Keep it light. High fat foods require a longer period to digest. A bowl of fiber cereal or half a tuna sandwich works for me.
> 2. Establish a step-by-step routine. Include a bath and a boring sitcom. Read a dull novel.
> 3. To catch up on sleep go to bed an hour early. Wake up at your normal time, even on weekends.
> 4. Your mattress should be firm, not hard. Shut your door, turn your telephone off, turn on your answering machine, close your eyes, and sleep.

In a recent study at the Sleep Laboratory at the University of Washington, exercisers not only improved their aerobic fitness by thirteen percent, they extended their deep sleep capabilities by thirty-three percent. Exercise especially improves sleep for those with low fitness levels and older adults.

Regardless of whether the exercise benefits sleep because of increased fatigue, elevated body temperature, or decreased stress, it works!

Martial Arts Cross-Training for Fitness

Martial arts cross-training is becoming increasingly popular. My martial arts cross-training program is designed to improve your martial arts performance.

Begin with a shadowboxing warm-up, followed by light stretching. Next perform a five minute abdominal routine, targeting your rectus abdominis, obliques, and transverse abdominis.

This serves as a warm up for weight training. Each day train a different muscle group. On Mondays work your back and biceps. Tuesdays, your chest and triceps. Wednesdays, your legs and shoulders. Never train a muscle group more than twice a week.

Following your weight training, perform a cardio-kickboxing bench aerobics routine. Vary the program daily.

At this point, your legs are sufficiently warmed, and you're ready for power plyometrics. Plyometrics consist of ten different jumping drills which enhance power. Then, jog and shuffle around the room, followed by combinations, kata, and sparring. Finish with heavy stretching and a cool-down.

Cross-Training/Machines. Your choice of workout machines are endless. The best indoor device is the one that you will utilize. Most end up as clothes hangers. If a product seems too good to be true it is. Infomercials lead you to believe you can burn one thousand calories in "just a few short minutes a day." Physically fit individuals may burn between 500 to 700 calories per hour, depending on the intensity of their exercise. Beware of contraptions that claim to spot reduce fat. There are no magic gadgets that "melt" fat from your thighs, hips, and waist.

Try before you buy. Some outlet stores allow you to work out in the store prior to making a purchase. Wear your warm up suit and test your favorite machine. Is it durable, comfortable, and solid? How does it feel on your knees and lower back? Can you maintain a neutral pelvis? Is the seat acceptable? Check the padding. Is it sturdy? What about noise levels? Will it fit in your home? Must you assemble it yourself?

Expect to spend a few hundred dollars for a machine that will last. Especially a treadmill. Inexpensive non-motorized units create an unnatural feel. A solid motorized treadmill will cost over a thousand dollars. An inclined one- or two-horsepower motorized treadmill will provide you the same intensity as jogging, without the high impact strain on your shins, back, and knees. Use the handrails to support your weight if you lose your balance. Otherwise keep your hands off the rails. When walking up a grade maintain perfect posture, with only a slight bend in your waist.

A reliable stationary bike is not as expensive as a quality treadmill. It is easy on your body and provides a tremendous cardiovascular workout. Purchase one that uses a friction belt such as the Keiser Power Pacer, or a model that functions on wind resistance such as the Schwinn Airdyne. Bypass bikes that use caliper brakes to raise the workload. These low budget versions make a smooth pedal stroke all but impossible. Adjust the seat so your knees are slightly bent on the downstroke. Use toe clips to pull as well as push to spin perfect little circles and increase your revolutions per minute (RPM's).

Other less popular home exercise devices include:
- Rowing machines—great for muscular endurance (Figure 5-2) but they're boring and require an unfamiliar movement.
- Cross-country ski machines—terrific total body workout but they tie up your hands so you cannot sip water or change channels on the television.
- Stair climbing machines—super for your legs, heart, and lungs but the good ones cost more than $2,000.
- Exercise riders—may be okay for beginners but they have been shown to damage knees and lower backs if used excessively.
- Medicine balls and rebounders—great for plyometric training (Figure 5-3).
- Torso machines—provide you with a safe and motivational training aid.

Kids Training

One third of all teenagers are inactive. Only thirty-two percent of kids aged six to seventeen meet minimum standards for cardiovascular fitness, flexibility, muscular strength, and endurance.

Forty percent of first graders have at least one coronary artery disease (CAD) risk factor. Thirty percent of all school aged children are at risk for CAD and premature death as adults.

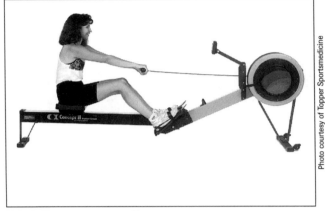

Figure 5-2

According to a *USA Today* poll, about twenty percent of children aged nine to eleven said they have been on a diet. Thirteen percent of adolescent boys, and twice that number of their female peers say they have dieted.

Since 1960 obesity increased fifty-four percent in elementary school children, and thirty-nine percent in high schoolers. Twenty five percent of all school aged children are obese. The longer kids are obese, the more likely they will remain so. Obese infants with obese parents are 2.5 times more likely to become obese adults. Obese adolescents have a ninety percent chance of becoming obese adults.

Poor heath practices tend to run in families. Your youngsters will adopt your habits. Involve your children in martial arts as early as possible. But don't work them out all day long. Kids are physiologically different than adults.

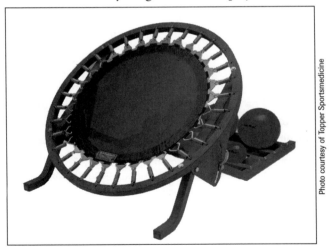

Figure 5-3

Before puberty children cannot keep up with adults. They have less muscle glycogen leading to a decreased ability to perform anaerobic tasks. They have a lower maximal and submaximal cardiac output. Their hearts are only thirty percent the size of yours. They carry less blood, therefore less oxygen is provided to fuel their punches and kicks.

Kids generally have low resting blood pressure. Similarly they have a low absolute VO_2 maximum (the amount of oxygen carried to the muscles per minute).

Your offspring have a quick-energy creatine phosphate system similar to yours. They have superior recovery rates, and they reach a steady state faster than you do.

Their bodies are well suited for martial arts. Your heirs have smaller lungs than you.

By the age of eight, your children's lungs are only twenty percent the size of yours. Their bones are smaller and more fragile. They lack carpal bones in the wrist. The ends of their bones are still growing and are vulnerable to injury. The epiphyseal plates of their radius and ulna bones (forearm bones), femur (thigh bone), tibia (shin bone), and fibula (small bone in the lower leg) stop growing in their late teens.

Youngsters are at a high risk for heat illness due to their immature cardiovascular systems, greater surface area, increased metabolic cost (more heat is produced), immature sweat glands (less sweat volume), and increased core temperature. Kids acclimatize slower. Because of this, the American Academy of Pediatrics (AAP) recommends to restrain intensity and duration initially, with a gradual increase over eleven to fourteen days.

Children should wear light weight absorbent clothing, no rubberized sweatsuits. And they should not rely on their thirst mechanism. Instead they should drink at least 150 milliliters of fluid every fifteen to thirty minutes during activity.

Overuse injuries are a concern. Be careful that children do not increase their frequency, intensity, or duration of martial arts activity drastically (ie. more than ten percent). Watch for strength and flexibility imbalances. Replace their footwear when appropriate. Look for misalignment of lower extremities.

The new AAP guidelines recommend that if children lift weights they should use high repetition, low resistance. Emphasize muscle balance, flexibility, and proper technique. Programs should be conducted by trained adults. And avoid weightlifting, power lifting, and body building until full sexual maturity.

Kids won't grow large muscles because they lack androgen-protein synthesis, which is not sufficient until adolescence. Boys and girls strength remain relatively equal until puberty.

Children should consume carbohydrates as fifty percent of their diet. Emphasize complex carbohydrates instead of simple sugars. Limit fast foods. Fifteen to twenty percent of their calories should come from protein. Insufficient protein could cause anemia and slowed growth. Thirty percent of daily calories should come from fat. Up until the age of two, infants and toddlers should consume whole milk. After age two they should drink 2% milk. And young adults can wean themselves to half percent or skim milk. Beyond age twelve, fats should comprise only twenty to thirty percent of their total calories.

Emphasize fun during your kids martial arts, not winning and hard work. Kids naturally enjoy martial arts, muscle strength and endurance training, flexibility work, and healthy nutrition. They will work out if they have fun and are allowed to be with their friends. You, as their parents are their greatest influence. Be kid-specific. Make martial arts exciting and easy to enjoy. Offer achievable goals. And challenge different abilities.

Older Adult Martial Arts Training Program

My unique mind/body fitness-conditioning program is for healthy, older adults who are looking for research-based, safe, and effective exercises to be in the best shape of their lives.

It is never too early to begin martial arts, and it is rarely, if ever too late. Begin slowly, progress gradually, and have realistic expectations. A study showed that older adults with the lowest scores for walking speed, balance, and ability to rise from a chair were nearly five times more likely to be disabled four years later compared to those who scored the highest.

Stiff muscles, joints, and lack of energy, sometimes called "aging pains" are actually "lack of activity" pains. When you lose your mobility, your self image decreases with your mood, and your sleep suffers.

Regular joint loading and movement are necessary to maintain cartilage function and joint range of motion. Reduced activity adversely affects the mechanical properties of cartilage. Martial arts increases capillary density and enzymatic activity.

Disuse accelerates negative changes that occur with aging. My program can slow or reverse age-related loss of strength, flexibility, and endurance.

As you become stronger and more flexible, you can do things you used to do. This may mean the difference between life in a chair and active adventure.

Older muscles are similar to younger ones, when asked to lift more, they become stronger. A sixty-eight year old on my program may function at a higher level than an eighteen year old. Older adults can increase strength as much as three hundred percent.

Follow the programs in this book and you will:
- Maintain and improve your cardiovascular fitness.
- Promote muscle strength, flexibility, and balance.
- Prevent or modify chronic disease.
- Prevent falls and fractures.
- Relieve anxiety, insomnia, and depression.
- Increase your social contacts.
- Care for yourself and increase your chances for an independent lifestyle.
- Improve your overall quality of life.
- Increase your metabolism.
- Lose fat.
- Increase your bone-mineral density.
- Increase your glucose uptake to help prevent diabetes.
- Manage your blood pressure.
- Improve your blood lipid levels (HDL-LDL cholesterol.)
- Decrease your low back pain and arthritis.
- Fight depression.
- Decrease your risk of injury.
- Increase your gastrointestinal transit time.
- Improve your posture. You will stand upright and appear younger.

My goal is to help you gain two pounds of muscle in two months. I want to strengthen your entire body, especially your back and neck.

Getting Older, Getting Better. Older adults are at risk for osteoporosis and bone fractures. Three high-risk areas include your lower spine, hips, and wrists.

Years ago if you acquired osteoporosis and were not feeling well, a physician might prescribe rest. Now doctors dictate exercise such as martial arts training.

Do not attempt to follow your grandchildren jumping off monkey bars and out of swings. You may have difficulty with eccentric contractions (jumping down and landing) and forceful movements.

Instead, strength training with the Sport Cord, dumbbells, or weight machines is beneficial. Lifting weights strengthens your bones. Your muscles pull on tendons that pull your bones. Proper nutrition and hormone levels mediate improvements in your bone density.

As you mature, you lose Type II B Fast Twitch muscle fibers. Your muscles tend to get weaker and smaller. Strength training reduces their rate of decline.

You can enhance your strength using a resistance program. The first phase of your improvement is due to neurological efficiency. You learn to recruit more muscle fibers. Sending signals from your brain to your muscles keeps your muscles activated.

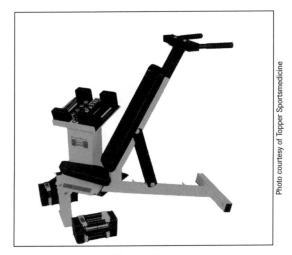

Photo courtesy of Topper Sportsmedicine

Figure 5-4

The second phase of your development stems from strengthened connective tissue. Tendons and ligaments become more powerful.

Young martial artists enjoy a third phase of advancement. Their testosterone kicks in. You probably will not experience testosterone elevation. Your strength will improve with little muscle enlargement.

You can increase muscle with resistance training, but you can't do much about losses in circulating anabolic hormones that increase muscle. Anabolic hormones increase protein synthesis. We lose fast twitch muscle fibers as we age. Fast twitch fibers are responsible for fast kicks. Bill Wallace is a world class anomaly by kicking fast into his fifties.

Strength training is extremely beneficial for your age group. One study showed that not only did lifting weights increase strength by fifty percent, but also subjects walking time improved by a significant factor. Strengthening muscles increased walking speed, regardless of aerobic condition.

Another study investigated the relationship between older adults and reaction time/movement time. Reaction time was designated by the amount of seconds it took for older adults to begin to respond to a stimulus. Movement time was the number of seconds from the initiation of effort until completion of the action. Subjects were instructed to walk normally through a pathway. When a light randomly blinked, subjects were required to stop and turn in one direction or the other. Results demonstrated that older adults had normal reaction time. Their movement time was compromised compared to their younger counterparts, however.

Roberta Rikli, Ph.D., professor of kinesiology, reported in the March 1994 issue of *Research Quarterly* that strong muscles reacted quicker than flabby ones. Forty-four women hit a footpad when a signal was given. Those with the strongest leg muscles reacted the fastest. Toned muscles have more nerve fibers and blood vessels to help the impulse get from thought to action.

Resistance training improves your balance. The heavier the weight, the better. But begin light. Gradually add weight. Be sure you can perform ten repetitions with perfect form before advancing to a heavier weight. Do not increase your resistance more than five percent in a single workout. If you do not have a set of weights with small, adjustable increments (Figure 5-4), perform more repetitions at your previous intensity. Most gyms have ten pound weight increments. After you can perform eighteen repetitions, increase the weight ten pounds.

> ## Weight training tips for the older adult:
>
> 1. The first eight weeks should employ minimum resistance to allow for your connective tissue to strengthen.
> 2. Emphasize proper technique and maintain your normal breathing.
> 3. Perform all of your exercises in a controlled manner. Never let the amount of weight dictate your form.
> 4. Your exercises should be performed in a range of motion that is pain free.
> 5. Perform multi-joint exercises (closed chain) as opposed to single joint exercises.
> 6. Your strength training should be performed regularly, not hit or miss.

Extend a dumbbell to the front of your body. Muscles in your back must counterbalance. Raise a weight from your side. Muscles on your other side brace your effort. Whenever you lift free weights, muscles throughout your body must stabilize your motion.

Consider older adults unfamiliar with weight training. They grasp five-pound sets of dumbbells and lift them to waist level. Their blood pressures rise, at first. If these individuals continue to strength train, their bodies gradually adapt and grow stronger. The stronger they become, the less their blood pressure increases upon physical demand. Soon, hoisting five-pound dumbbells affects their blood pressure as if they were plucking a blade of grass.

Longevity. Well-conditioned hearts deliver more blood and nutrients to muscles, increasing their ability to work. There is less chance for blood clots decreasing the chances for heart attack and stroke.

And you are not required to kick and punch for hours to receive cardiovascular benefits. Steven Blair, PED of the Cooper Clinic in Dallas suggests that a daily half-hour workout should put you in the fit zone.

You may work out too much, however. High level training can destroy red blood cells. During a 2,100 kilometer, sixteen day relay run, men in their sixties and seventies experienced a twenty percent loss in red blood cells.

Aging reduces the elasticity of lung tissue, stiffens the chest wall, lessens the strength of muscles used in breathing, and increases airway resistance. Breathing requires a higher percentage of energy. If you train in the martial arts, the muscles and lung tissue expand so you may inhale and exhale with the same ease and vigor as you did when you were in your twenties.

Martial arts training makes your brain more alert and quicker. In the March, 1996 issue of *Research Quarterly for Exercise and Sport* a study demonstrated that when people watched a fifteen minute informational video during exercise, their brain waves were more active than when they viewed the video from a lounge chair.

Activity has been shown to increase I.Q. in the elderly. Martial arts training improves mood and wards off depression. Whether these changes are due to increased circulation, adrenaline production, or some other factor is unclear.

Physical fitness is worth forty years in helping an aging body transport oxygen. A fit seventy year old may have better oxygen carrying capacity than a sedentary thirty-five year old.

Inactivity has recently been reported as a risk factor as debilitat-

Strength training tips for the older adult:

- Machine weights are preferred over free weights for older adults.
- When returning from a layoff, use a resistance that is less than 50 percent of the previous intensity, and gradually increase the resistance.
- Strength training should be performed year round and not on a hit or miss basis.
- Wear proper foot wear (good traction/proper cushioning).
- Avoid all jerky, rapid twisting or turning of any body part.
- Avoid excessive compression of the abdominal area.
- Avoid bending all the way over at the waist.
- Avoid standing on one leg for longer than eight counts.
- Do not lift your chin past neutral and drop your head back. This can cause cervical compression and dizziness.
- Avoid dropping your arms forcefully from a position above your head or out to the sides. After lifting the shoulders up, the return to neutral should be slow and controlled.
- Alternate finger work with wrist work in order to prevent over-stressing potentially inflamed joints.
- Avoid forcefully twisting from side to side.
- Keep your back in a neutral position; your spine relaxed up against the back of a chair to allow for more freedom of movement from the hip socket.
- Whenever your legs are extended to the front, be sure that you keep your abdominal muscles engaged and back straight with no hyperextension of the lower back.
- If you perform push-ups, avoid flexing the elbows more than ninety degrees.
- Do not perform wall sits if you are unsteady or have very weak quadriceps.

ing as smoking. Exercisers who smoke, have high cholesterol, and high blood pressure are better off than non-exercisers who do not have these risk factors according to the July 17th, 1996 issue of the *Journal of the American Medical Association.*

Eating high fat foods combined with a sedentary lifestyle is a disaster for your arteries. And when you add that to a stressful job, your chances for heart disease skyrocket. Risk factors for coronary artery disease (CAD) include:

- Age: men older than forty-five. Women older than fifty-five.
- Blood pressure: 140/90 or greater.
- Cigarette smoking: more than four cigarettes a day.
- Diabetes: type I (juvenile) or type II (adult).
- Elevated Cholesterol: LDL greater than 160. HDL less than 35.
- Family History of CAD. Premature cardiovascular disease.
- Gross Inactivity. If you train less than twice a week.

Your body was not designed to sit for long periods. Sitting places pressure on your back. Especially if you are not conscious of your posture. You sit all day long. You sit in your car, at your desk, at lunch, dinner, and after dinner on your favorite recliner watching martial arts flicks.

Nearly one million Americans die each year from cardiovascular disease. Americans suffer 1.25 million coronary events annually. Twenty-five percent of these deaths are from coronary artery disease (CAD), of which atherosclerosis is the primary cause. CAD is the leading cause of death in this country.

Plaque in the arteries is thought to occur from disturbances to the endothelium (inner lining of the artery). This damage can occur from smoking and high blood pressure (hypertension). Once this destruction occurs, individuals with elevated cholesterol are prone to plaque buildup.

Treatment options such as by-pass surgery and angioplasty are common. Three hundred thousand patients per year endure bypass surgery, and a similar number undergo angioplasty.

Non invasive medications include beta blockers and calcium channel blockers. Lifestyle changes include diet, martial arts training, and mind/body techniques to decrease stress.

Eating For Life. Fruits and vegetables contain health-promoting, disease-busting chemicals. In fact, "phyto" means plant. Phytochemicals are in salads, tomato sauce, and vegetable stir-fry. Just about any vegetable contains some type of phytochemical.

Your backyard garden has some of the best protection against heart disease and cancer. You do not require a green thumb to grow tomatoes. Tomatoes have been shown to contain thousands of phytochemicals.

Lycopene, present in tomato sauce, is an antioxidant. Antioxidants help prevent heart disease, prostate, and stomach cancer.

Antioxidants can be likened to samurai warriors. They prevent free electrons from ravaging your system. Free electrons, commonly called free radicals, increase oxidation, "rusting" your organs. Antioxidants bind with free radicals and destroy them. In so doing, antioxidants themselves are sacrificed.

Another group of antioxidants are carotenes. Carotenes give carrots their orange color. Yams, sweet potatoes, green leafy vegetables, peaches, cantaloupe, and apricots contain carotenes.

Chives, leeks, onions, shallots, and garlic contain sulfides. If you can side step their pungent aroma, garlic and onions can aid in preventing stomach and colon cancer.

Eating broccoli, brussels sprouts, cauliflower, turnips, watercress, kohlrabi, and cabbage is a natural way to reduce your risk of lung and stomach cancer.

Soy is a phytoestrogen. Phytoestrogens suppress estrogen. Estrogen is a hormone-dependent cancer. Soy may help prevent breast cancer and prostate cancer. Other soy foods include tempeh, miso, and tofu.

Green tea has a type of antioxidant called a polyphenol. Polyphenols may be protective against stomach, skin, and lung cancer.

Vitamin E is probably the most well known antioxidant. And vitamin E is also a phytochemical. Vegetable oils contain alpha linoleic acid, a huge source of vitamin E. Vitamin E helps to defend against muscle cell membrane damage. If you regularly endure vigorous martial arts workouts, vitamin E helps manage muscle inflammation.

The latest research suggests we should attempt to get our phytochemicals and antioxidants from foods rather than pills. Supplement manufacturers have not as yet found a way to extract all of the possible benefits from phytochemicals and grind them into tablets.

Aging Painlessly: Older Adult Resistance Training Tips. Include at least one resistance exercise for all major muscle groups including quadriceps (thighs), hamstrings (back of thighs), gluteals (hips), pectorals (chest), latissimus (back), deltoids (shoulders), trapezius and rhomboids (upper back), abdominals (stomach), and erector spinae (back).

Ideally each training session should be completed within thirty minutes. Sessions lasting longer than sixty minutes may have a detrimental effect on exercise adherence.

The first eight weeks you should employ minimum resistance to allow for connective tissue adaptation. Emphasize proper technique and maintain normal breathing.

Initial overload should be achieved by increasing the number of repetitions, and later by increasing the weight. All exercises should be performed in a controlled manner, never using a resistance that would prohibit you from completing at least eight repetitions.

Exercises should be performed in a range of motion that is pain free. Perform one set of eight to twelve repetitions with a specific weight that elicits a perceived exertion rating of "somewhat hard."

If you are an older martial artist, be aware of a few modifications in your training program. Your vision, hearing, and reaction time may decrease. Your strength and endurance functional capacity may lessen, causing you to lose muscle mass and reduce your aerobic capacity.

But that does not mean older adult martial artists should throw in the towel. In fact the opposite is true. A recent study demonstrated that men and women in their eighties and nineties improved their strength 150 percent on a sixteen week weight training program. Many walked without their canes, and stood up from a seated position without assistance. It is well documented that elite martial artists train well into their twilight years.

Balance may be improved by using the following exercises taken from the November, 1995 issue of *American Health:*

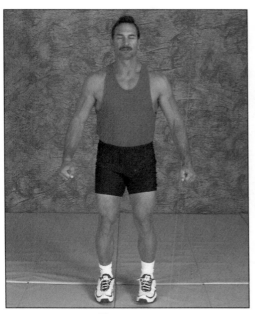

Figure 5-5

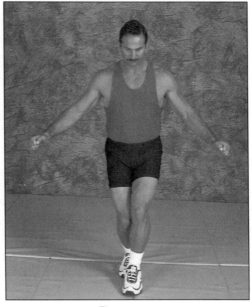

Figure 5-6

1. Toe stand: Rise up on your toes, hold for ten seconds (Figure 5-5).
   Week One: one hand for support.
   Week Two: No hands.
   Week Three: Eyes closed/no hands.

2. Tandem Stand: One foot in front/touching heel-toe (Figure 5-6).
   Week One: One hand for support.
   Week Two: No hands.
   Week Three: Eyes closed/no hands.

3. One-Legged Stand: Stand on one leg (Figure 5-7).
   Week One: One hand for support.
   Week Two: No hands.
   Week Three: Eyes closed/no hands.

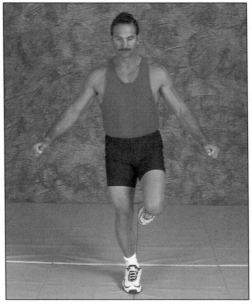

Figure 5-7

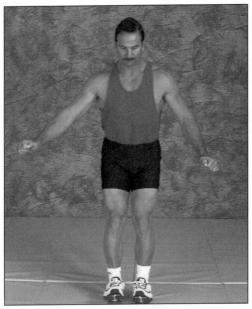

Figure 5-8

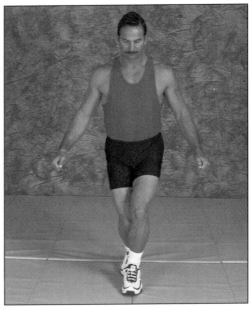

Figure 5-9

4. Heel Stand: Balance on heels (Figure 5-8).
   Week One: One hand for support.
   Week Two: No hands.
   Week Three: Eyes closed/no hands.

5. Toe Walk: Walk while on tiptoes down the hall (Figure 5-9).
   Week One: One hand for support.
   Week Two: No hands.

6. Tandem Forward Walk: One foot in front of the other/ walk down the hall (Figure 5-10).
   Week One: One hand for support.
   Week Two: No hands.

7. Heel Walk: Walk while heels down the hall (Figure 5-11).
   Week One: One hand for support.
   Week Two: No hands.

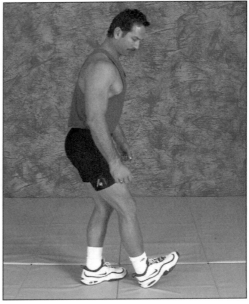

Figure 5-10

8. Tandem Backward Walk: Walk backwards toe to heel (Figure 5-12).
   Week One: One hand for support.
   Week Two: No hands.

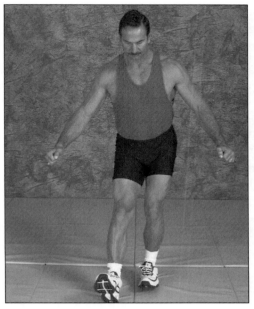

Figure 5-11

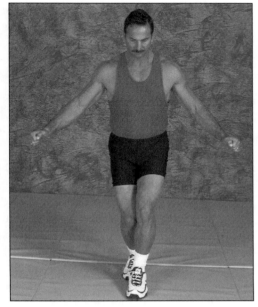

Figure 5-12

Home Remedies

There is more to martial arts training than demonstrating your genetic giftedness. Pacing is extremely important to exemplary martial arts performance. Knowing when to turn it on and when to rest can help you enjoy your martial art, reach optimal physical condition, and be your best. The hard part is distinguishing overtraining from laziness.

Pay attention to nagging injuries. Problem areas for martial artists include backs, knees, shoulders, and elbows. To protect your back strengthen your abdominals, leg, hips, and stretch your hamstrings. Your knees can be reinforced by strengthening your quadriceps and your hamstrings. Stretch and strengthen your shoulders. To prevent tendinitis in your elbows, strengthen your forearms.

If you incur a soft tissue injury be prepared for a longer recovery than when you were a teenager. A simple muscle strain may result in a debilitating back problem. An irritated elbow may evolve into tendinitis.

My martial arts training lead to a variety of injuries. Sprains and strains required rest, ice, and elevation. Multiple shin and forearm contusions healed by themselves. I have received a number of concussions. One of these precipitated a retinal tear in my left eye. My retinal tear was diagnosed during a mandatory pre-fight eye exam. My only symptom was "floaters" so the opthamologist suggested no treatment. He did not allow me to fight the following week, but he did refer me to an otolaryngologist to straighten my deviated septum. Years ago doctors "packed" the upper nostrils. When I returned a week following my rhinoplasty operation for my follow up appointment, the doctor removed the packing. Either I was not told, or I forgot that there was packing up my nose. But it was the most enjoyably painful experience I can recall.

Injuries are a part of life. Especially as we mature. Eighty percent of our ailments will heal themselves. Doctors and chiropractors can help us through the rest of our maladies. But if an injury persists more than a few days, seek professional help. Ask your doctor about some of my home remedies below.

Plantar fascitis, an excruciating pain on the bottom of your foot near your heel is crippling. It is an inflammation of the plantar fascia, a ligament running across the bottom of the foot. It hurts especially upon stepping out of bed in the morning.

I first developed plantar fascitis during international martial arts competitions. In those days plantar fascitis was labeled a heel spur. Although my X-rays were clear, the pain was excruciating in the heels of both feet. The diagnosis was inflammation of the tendons on the bottoms of my heels. They were routinely treated with cortisone injections. Every six months I visited my doctor and watched him stick an enormous needle into my heel. It hurt "so good" because I knew by the next day I would be pain free for six months. Since then treatment has changed. First your foot is taped with a pad to support the arch. If pain diminishes, your doctor fashions an orthotic to fit comfortably within your shoe.

Shin splints, a debilitating ache on the front of the shins frequently sidelined me in high school and college. Stretching the calf muscles helped, and so did curtailing activity. Once the pain subsided, I found an exercise that prevented shin splints from recurring. Sit on the edge of a bench and hook the handle of a bucket onto the top of your foot. Slowly flex and extend your ankle, strengthening the anterior tibialis muscle on the front of your shin. Do ten repetitions with each foot once a day for the first week. The second week, perform two sets of ten repetitions every other day. Thereafter, complete three sets of ten repetitions twice a week.

Low back pain will strike one out of three of us sometime in our lives. The method I use to prevent its painful reappearance is a combination of ice, stretching, and strengthening. I stretch my hamstrings (the back of my legs) daily, and perform abdominal and leg strengthening exercises a few times a week. I'm also careful to use my legs instead of my back when shoveling or lifting.

Knee pain can be frightening. You might be walking and unexplainably your knees weaken and buckle. Or you bend to lift a heavy object and a sharp pain precedes your collapse. Pedaling a stationary bike is a natural, easy way to strengthen the quadriceps muscle surrounding the knee. Although your knee joint may be painful, strengthening the adjoining muscles will support your movement. After your quadriceps are stronger, try some light leg extensions on a weight machine. Or you can sit on the edge of a bench and hook a bucket handle to your ankle and flex and extend your leg. Perform the same set and repetition program as presented in the shin splint section above.

Achilles tendinitis never was a problem for me until I traveled to Florida for vacation. I enjoyed running the beach, but each day the back of my heel was sore. One morning it was so painful I could not walk. I finally realized that the sand was allowing my foot to flex further than it normally does on hard ground. Recovery was slow. I minimized activities such as rope jumping and tennis. I took the advice of a friend and inserted a heel pad into my shoe. The pad lifted my foot slightly, taking the pressure off my achilles tendon. Two months later I was jogging comfortably.

Shoulder pain was a nuisance during high school and college tennis. In those days, weight training was not recommended as performance enhancing. Especially for a skill sport such as tennis. But during my sophomore year at Penn State I enrolled in a weight training course. Within a few months my shoulder pain diminished. I have continued weight training since. So have Andre Agassi, Martina Navratilova, and most other professional tennis players. When shoulder pain recurs I use dumbbells rather than a straight bar. Dumbbells allow an individualized range of motion to work around soreness.

Hip pain never was a concern until recently. The top of my hip, just below my waist, hurt so badly I was forced to limp. Then I remembered a hip stretch I read in *The Physician and Sports Medicine*. Stand with your left hand on a wall with your feet less than shoulder width apart. Cross your left foot over your right keeping both knees slightly bent. Lean to your right bending slightly from your waist. Repeat on your other side. I perform this stretch daily for both hips. I hold the stretch for three seconds. I have not experienced hip pain since beginning this program.

Low blood sugar may be a problem that you are not consciously aware of. Symptoms for me included mid-morning and mid-afternoon fatigue and irritability. I thought these feelings were unavoidable until I consumed a small protein-carbohydrate snack at 10:00 A.M. and 3:00 P.M. I immediately noticed an increase in energy and performance. I was less hungry at lunch and dinner. Now it is a habit to eat three meals and two snacks daily. For me snacks include fruit, cereal, yogurt, or a sandwich.

Conclusion

A martial artist's resting heart rate is generally slower than a sedentary person's. In fact a martial artist usually has a stronger heart, providing for a greater stroke volume, to eject more blood through the body with each beat.

Not surprisingly, to me martial arts is a fountain of youth. In fact I believe working out is the future of preventive medicine. Martial arts can strengthen joints, improve moods, and prevent coronary artery disease. Soon doctors will be prescribing workouts just as they prescribe medicine.

Martial artists take responsibility to learn about their bodies. Some are concerned about what they eat. They try alternative approaches such as acupuncture and herbal remedies. Holistic programs treat the whole person rather than specific symptoms. Living a long and healthy existence has a great deal to do with lifestyle.

In the cost-cutting world of health maintenance organizations (HMO's), martial arts is an inexpensive intervention technique. Used in conjunction with a doctor's recommendations, martial arts can improve the quantity and quality of your life.

Be sure to warm up before you work out. This simply means to begin martial arts slowly and progress gradually, rather than jump kicking out the door. Some experts recommend stretching both before and after training. But if you only have time for a single stretching routine, elongate your muscles after they are warm from a vigorous martial arts workout.

Drink water every chance you get. If not, your blood volume decreases and your exercise performance will decline. Drink before, during, and after your workout. Your urine should be clear if you are fully hydrated.

Always anticipate your martial arts training. If you feel tired, bored, sluggish, and your heart rate is high, you may be overtraining. Take a day off once in a while and be sure you are getting enough sleep. As you mature you need more rest between training sessions.

Back aches, knee problems, shin, and foot ailments may be the result of wearing improper footwear. Be sure your shoes have proper cushioning and fit your feet. They should have a durable outer sole, and firm insole. Replace your shoes after six months.

Place your right hand on your stomach and your left hand on your chest. Breathe so that only your right hand moves. When you breathe from your stomach, your diaphragm is activated. This allows you to take deeper and longer breaths, using more of your lung capacity for exercise.

Martial arts is stress to your body. If you are unhealthy or disease ridden, it is not advisable to begin a training program. Instead, check with your doctor and wait until you recover. If you are healthy, begin your regimen slowly. Most folks do too much too soon and end up hurting themselves. That is the reason less than fifty percent of beginning martial artists continue to workout after three months.

When you are attempting to improve your martial arts, take it easy. Increase your intensity only five percent at a time. Any more than this small increment may lead to injury. Ex-high school/college athletes are notorious for attempting flying spinning back kicks the first day of training.

An-All Purpose Strength and Safe Plyometric Program for All Athletes

A monthlong, three times a week (Monday, Wednesday, Friday) workout with one set of most every exercise.

Explosive Movements

Squat Thrust: Stand with your feet shoulder-width apart. In one fluid motion, while keeping your feet flat on the ground, squat until your thighs are parallel to the ground (no farther) and place your palms flat on the floor alongside your feet. Keeping your weight planted over your arms, kick your feet straight back so that you end up in a straight-armed push-up position. Do one push-up, hop back into the starting squat, and stand (Figures A-1 to A-5).

Week 1: 20 reps
Week 2: 30 reps
Week 3: 40 reps
Week 4: 60 reps

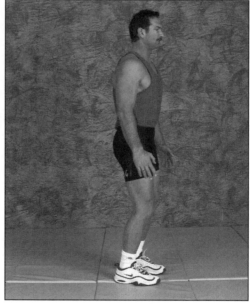

Figure A-1

Stair Sprint: If your training area has enough room, sprint fifteen to twenty yards to the base of a flight of stairs, then sprint up them. Take the stairs two or three at a time, raising your knees high. Try not to hunch your torso forward, and stop if you experience any lower-back pain.

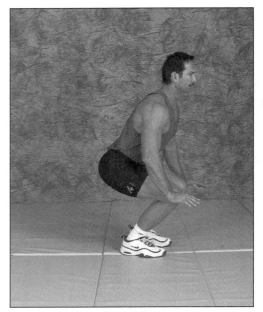

Figure A-2

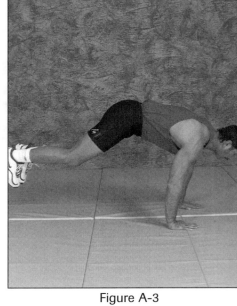

Figure A-3

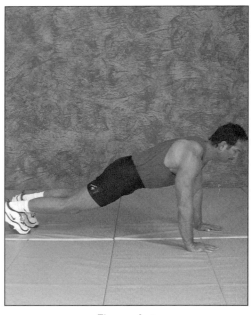

Figure A-4

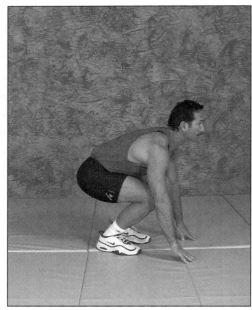

Figure A-5

Week 1: 2 sprints
Week 2: 4 sprints
Week 3: 4 sprints
Week 4: 6 sprints

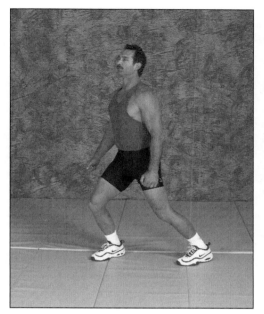

Figure A-6

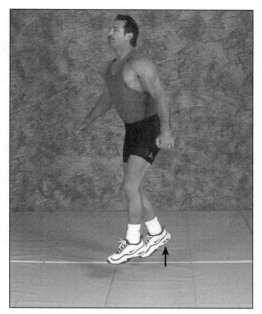

Figure A-7

Lunge Jump: With your head up and back in its natural alignment, step forward with your left leg, lowering your body until your front knee is bent ninety degrees and your right knee almost touches the floor. From this starting position, jump up a few inches and switch feet in the air, landing in the starting position with your right foot forward (Figures A-6 to A-8).

Week 1: 10 reps
Week 2: 15 reps
Week 3: 15 reps
Week 4: 20 reps

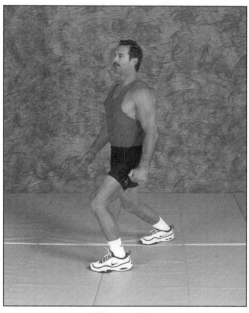

Figure A-8

Knee Up: Drive your right knee into the air toward your chest while simultaneously jumping up with your left leg. Bring your left knee up toward your chest while straightening your right knee to land. Switch legs and repeat.

Week 1: 6 reps
Week 2: 10 reps
Week 3: 16 reps
Week 4: 30 reps

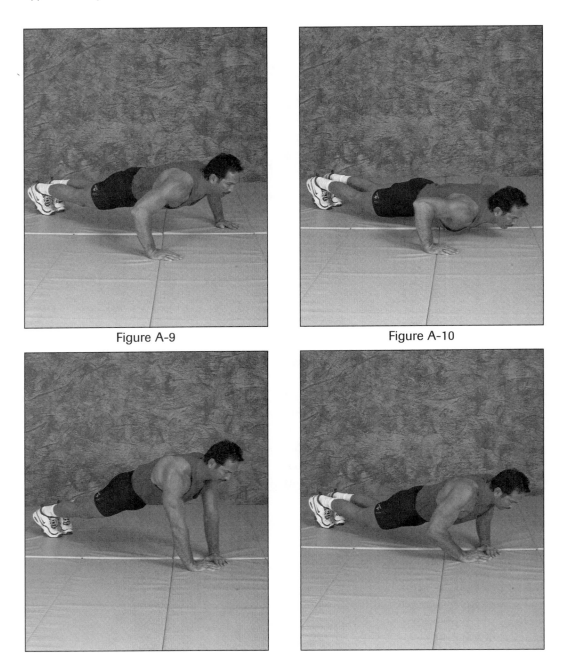

Figure A-9

Figure A-10

Figure A-11

Figure A-12

Upper Body Movements

Push-Up: Use the standard, back-straight military push-up form, but change grip position on each set. Start with a grip that is wider than your shoulders, then move to a shoulder's width grip and, finally, a "diamond" grip with your hands together and your thumbs and index fingers forming the diamond (Figures A-9 to A-13).

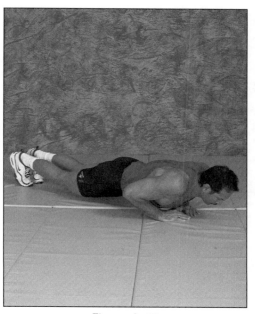

Figure A-13

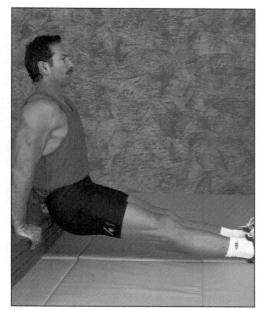

Figure A-14

Week 1: 20/15/10 reps
Week 2: 30/25/20 reps
Week 3: 40/35/30 reps
Week 4: 50/45/35 reps

Plyometric Push-Up: Follow the same form for a medium-grip push-up, but explode off the ground an inch or so at the end of each rep. Land softly, lower your chest to the ground slowly, then push yourself off the floor again. This will build explosiveness, but if you push yourself too hard, too soon, you'll face plant. Watch out.

Week 1: 6 reps
Week 2: 8 reps
Week 3: 10 reps
Week 4: 15 reps

Chair Dip: Place your hands on two chairs or a bench so that they are slightly behind your torso. You feet should rest on the floor or a bench two or three feet away. Your torso should be bent about ninety degrees at the waist. Lower your upper body as far as is comfortable, then push back up to the starting position (Figures A-14 to A-16).

Week 1: 30 reps
Week 2: 40 reps
Week 3: 50 reps
Week 4: 50 reps

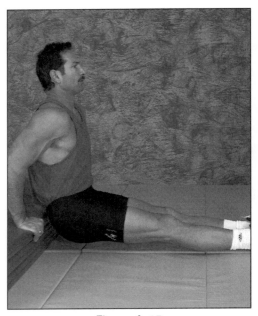

Figure A-15

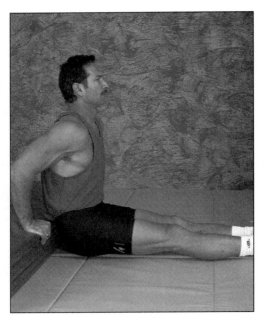

Figure A-16

Pull-Up: Grab the bar with your hands shoulder's width apart and slowly raise yourself as high as you can. Stop at the bottom of each repetition, but don't lock your arms. Keep your abdominals contracted, and your torso still at all times. Don't kip, and don't use momentum. (If you can easily do more than twelve pull-ups in a row, widen your grip and/or add resistance by wearing a weight belt or holding a dumbbell between your feet.)

Week 1: max. with perfect form
Week 2: max. with perfect form
Week 3: max. with perfect form
Week 4: max. with perfect form

Lower Body Movements

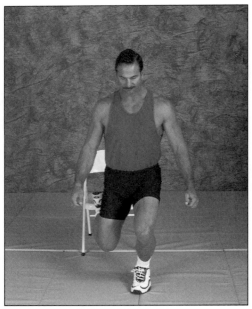

Figure A-17

One-Legged Squats: Stand six to twelve inches in front of a chair. Bend the knee of the non-working leg; support it on the chair. Squat deeply with the working leg, bending its knee about eighty degrees. Rise up until the knee is bent slightly (twenty degrees); do not lock your knee. Each rep should take several seconds—the idea is to move slowly through a full range of motion. (Figures A-17 to A-21)

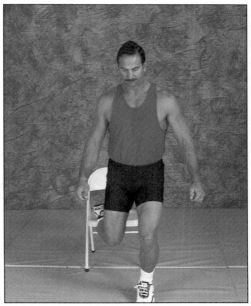

Figure A-18

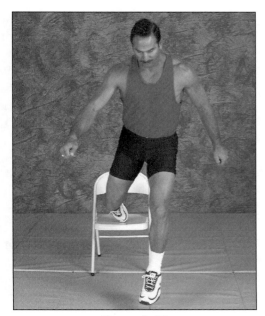

Figure A-19

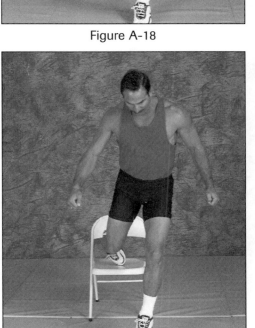

Figure A-20

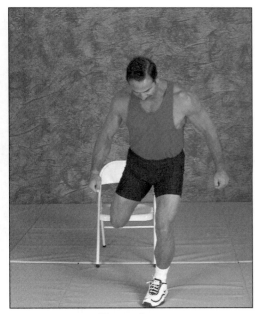

Figure A-21

Week 1: 25 reps per leg
Week 2: 30 reps per leg
Week 3: 35 reps per leg
Week 4: 40 reps per leg

Plie Squat: Stand with your feet slightly farther than shoulder's width apart; point the toes of both feet off to the sides at about a forty-five degree angle. Bend your knees until your core is directly over your heels. Then rise up on the balls of your feet, raising your heels; hold for an instant, then lower them slowly to the floor.

Week 1: 25
Week 2: 30
Week 3: 35
Week 4: 40

Lunge with Back Leg Lift: Start in a standard lunge position, then lift your back leg off the ground a few inches by contracting your glutes. Balance for a second, lower and repeat. Switch legs (Figure A-22).

Week 1: 10/leg
Week 2: 20/leg
Week 3: 25/leg
Week 4: 30/leg

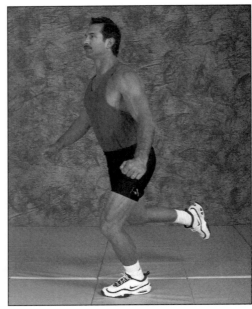

Figure A-22

Abdominal Movements

Butterfly Crunches: Lie on your back with your hands behind your head, then press the soles of your feet together a few inches in front of your groin. Wait a few seconds for your inner-thigh muscles to relax, then curl your torso a few inches toward your knees while

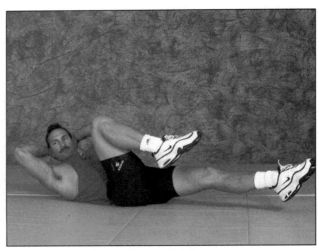

Figure A-23

keeping your lower back flat on the floor. Hold the contraction for a beat, then lower your shoulders. The physiologists like this variation because it focuses the entire contraction on your abs, not your hip muscles.

Week 1: 3 sets, 15 reps
Week 2: 3 sets, 25 reps
Week 3: 3 sets, 40 reps
Week 4: 3 sets, 50 reps

Twist Crunch: Lie on your back with your hands behind your head and your knees bent perpendicular to the floor. Crunch your torso forward while aiming your right elbow at your left knee; simultaneously extend your right leg in front of you. Slowly lower yourself back to the ground while returning your right leg to the starting position. Repeat on the opposite side, crunching your left elbow toward your right knee while extending your left leg. This will make your hip flexors ache, but for athletes, that's not a bad thing (Figures A-23 to A-24).

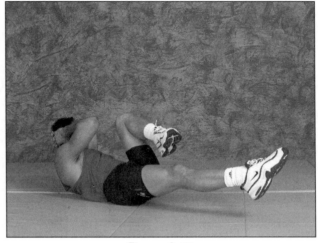

Figure A-24

Week 1: 3 sets, 15
Week 2: 3 sets, 20
Week 3: 3 sets, 25
Week 4: 3 sets, 30

Superman: Lie on your stomach with your arms straight out in front of you. Lift your arms and legs a few inches off the ground simultaneously until you feel your back muscles fully contract. Hold the tension for a few seconds, then slowly lower your legs and arms (Figures A-25).

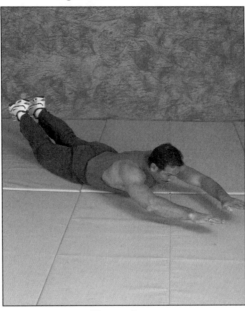

Week 1: 10 reps
Week 2: 10 reps
Week 3: 12 reps
Week 4: 15 reps

Figure A-25

Suggested Readings

Anderson, B, 1980. *Stretching.* Bolinas, California: Shelter Publication.

Benson, H. 1984. *Beyond the Relaxation Response.* New York: Times Books.

Benson, H. 1987. *Your Maximum Mind.* New York: Times Books.

Benson, H. 1993. *The Wellness Book.* New York: Simon & Schuster.

Borysenko, J. 1988. *Minding the Body, Mending the Mind.* New York: Bantam Books.

Csikszentmihalyi, M. 1994. *Flow: the Psychology of Optimal Experience.* New York: Simon & Schuster.

Edwards, S. 1993. *The Heart Rate Monitor Book.* Port Washington, New York: Polar Electro.

Dossey, Larry. 1993. *Healing Words.* New York: Harper Collins.

Freidman, M. 1989. "A master of moving meditation." *New Realities.* June. pp. 11-20.

Goleman, D. 1993. *Mind Body Medicine.* Yonkers, NY: Consumer Reports Books.

Langer, E. l989. *Mindfulness.* New York: Addison Wesley Pub. Co.

Lee, W., *Chinese Fitness,* 1997. Boston: YMAA Publication Center.

McKenzie R: *Treat Your Own Back,* ed 6. Waikanae, New Zealand: Spinal Publications, 1996.

Seabourne, T.G., 1998. *The Martial Arts Athlete—Mental and Physical Conditioning for Peak Performance.* Boston: YMAA Publication Center.

Seabourne, T.G. 1996. *Cross-Training.* Dubuque, Iowa: Eddie Bowers.

Seabourne, T.G., Weinberg, R.S., and Jackson, A. 1981. "Effects of visuo-motor behavior rehearsal, relaxation and imagery on karate performance." *Journal of Sport Psychology.* Vol. 3. no. 3. pp. 228-238

Seabourne, T.G., Weinberg, R.S., and Jackson, A., 1985. "Effect of arousal and relaxation instructions prior to the use of imagery." *Journal of Sport Behavior.* pp. 209-219

Wilmore, J., and Costill D. 1994. *Physiology of Sport and Exercise.* Champaign, Illinois: Human Kinetics Publishers.

Yang, J.M., 1999. *Classical Yang Style Taijiquan.* Boston: YMAA Publication Center.

Yang, J.M., 1998. *Back Pain—Chinese Qigong for Healing and Prevention.* Boston: YMAA Publication Center.

Glossary

Abdominal Fat Stress releases epinephrine, which reacts with hormone sensitive lipase, to help you lose fat around your waist. Too bad that doesn't work for fat around your hips.

Abdominals Flat, bandlike, muscles on the front of your trunk. They connect your pelvis to your rib cage.

Abductors A.K.A. outer thigh. These muscle includes your tensor fascia latae.

Acclimatization If you train in the heat, you get better at conserving sodium (salt). Your sweat is more dilute. You preserve sodium. If you lose too much sodium it is more difficult for you to remain hydrated.

Acetylcholine A neurotransmitter that slows your heart rate. It is controlled by your parasympathetic nervous system.

Active Isolated (AI) Stretching A type of stretching where you contract your antagonist muscle for two seconds prior to stretching your agonist for two seconds. You can do as many as ten repetitions of each stretch. The purpose of AI stretching is to inhibit the stretch reflex.

Active Recovery Toxins accumulate in your muscles after exercise. These waste products are drastically reduced if you perform some type of activity after your workout. Walking, pedaling, or light jogging for ten to fifteen minutes will greatly improve the breakdown of metabolites to reduce unwanted stiffness and soreness.

Acute Urinary Retention An enlarged prostate causes an inability to squeeze urine past it. Usually a catheter is required to transfer urine from the bladder to the urethra.

Adductors A.K.A. inner thigh. These muscles include your adductor magnus, adductor longus, adductor brevis, and gracilis.

Adipose Tissue A.K.A. fat. This is a yellowish substance within your fat cells. Years ago it was valuable during times of starvation. In over-fed America, adipose tissue around your waist and hips is a curse.

Aerobic Exercise Aerobic means "with oxygen." Move your large muscle groups in a rhythmic fashion and you are doing aerobics. Walking, jogging, stairclimbing, swimming, and jumping rope are examples.

Aerophagia Swallowing too much air.

Age-Related Macular Degeneration The part of your retina that is responsible for sharp, in-focus vision is called your macula. As you get older, your macula deteriorates.

Agonist The muscle group you are referring to.

Alcohol Moderate drinking is associated with a lower risk for heart disease in some individuals. One drink per day was found to increase the level of high-density lipoprotein (HDL) cholesterol, a.k.a. "good cholesterol," in your blood. The higher your HDL levels, the lower your risk for heart disease.

Aldosterone Your adrenal gland secretes this hormone. It is responsible for signaling your kidneys to conserve sodium and water. This raises your plasma volume. It raises your blood pressure too.

Alimentary Canal Another word for your gastrointestinal (GI) tract.

Allergies Allergies occur when your immune system reacts to pollen, mold, or dust. Your body perceives these irritants as if they were alien invaders. Your symptoms include watery nasal discharge; sneezing; coughing; itchy eyes, nose, and throat; nasal congestion; and dark circles under your eyes.

Alpha State A brain wave pattern characterized by relaxed concentration.

Alternative Approaches Dr. Dean Ornish has shown that patients may reverse their heart disease with a combination of a low-fat diet, meditation, and exercise. Norman Cousins healed his ankylosing spondylitis (a form of arthritis of the spine) by watching funny movies and high doses of vitamin C. Many patients have cured their digestive disturbances by avoiding certain foods.

Altitude Training The latest research suggests it is better to live at thirty-five hundred meters and train at fifteen hundred meters, then equivalent sea level training or equivalent altitude training. This flies in the face of previous research that suggested it was better to train at a higher altitude than the subsequent competition.

Amino Acids Amino acids are the building blocks of protein. You need not spend your hard earned money purchasing amino acid supplements. Instead eat lean proteins such as egg whites, chicken breast, turkey breast, fish, non-fat dairy, and game meats. Eight essential amino acids must be provided from your food. Non-essential amino acids are made within your body.

Amygdala This is the part of your brain that is involved with emotion and memory.

Amylase An enzyme that is secreted by your pancreas. It helps you digest carbohydrates.

Anaerobic Exercise Anaerobic means "without oxygen." High intensity, short duration activities are anaerobic. Weight training, sprinting, basketball, racketball, and tennis are anaerobic.

Androgens These are your male steroid hormones. They are produced in your adrenal glands and ovaries in women. These are the types of steroids that help you to build muscle.

Anemia Your body uses iron to make red blood cells. If your iron levels drop, then your body loses its ability to manufacture red blood cells. The fewer red blood cells you have, the less hemoglobin. As your hemoglobin drops, the ability of your blood to carry oxygen decreases and you have less energy. Symptoms of anemia include fatigue, shortness of breath, dizziness, light-headedness, fainting, and decreased resistance to colds and other infections.

Aneurysm This is a large bubble or pocket in your blood vessel. It is a weak spot in your vessel wall. If an aneurysm ruptures, it is life threatening.

Angina Chest pain that occurs when your heart does not get enough blood and oxygen from your coronary arteries. Your pain may be referred to your chest, jaw, arm, or a variety of other places. The pain can be sharp, dull, or a pressing sensation. Angina may last minutes or weeks.

Ankle Strengthening Place your foot on the floor against the leg of a chair. Push your foot against the chair sideways, both to the inside and outside, to strengthen the muscles that turn your ankle in and out. Try this—keep your heel planted. Move the front of your foot out sideways and back. When your ankle is strong enough, use a towel for resistance.

Ankylosing Spondylitis This is an inflammation of your spinal tissue. It is so painful it may lead to stiffness. This may cause you to change your posture and change the way your facets of your spine sit atop one another.

Annulus Fibrosus This is the protective, layered, outer portion of each of your spinal disks.

Antagonist The opposite of the muscle group you are referring to. For example the antagonist to the biceps is your triceps.

Antioxidants These are vitamins and minerals, including C, E, and beta carotene, zinc, selenium, and others, that are suggested to inhibit oxygen-based free radicals from attaching to and destroying your healthy organs and tissues.

Aorta This is the main artery that carries blood away from your heart.

Aphasia Difficulty speaking or understanding language. It usually occurs after a stroke. Aphasia affects the left hemisphere of the brain, where language is processed.

Apolipoproteins These are the proteins that combine with cholesterol and triglycerides. The combination is called lipoproteins.

Appendicitis Appendicitis is an acute inflammation of your appendix. Your appendix is a thin, tube-shaped structure that protrudes from the first section of your large intestine. Your appendix can become inflamed because of an anatomical obstruction, or a blockage of hardened feces. This inflammation can rapidly develop into an infection.

Aqueous Humor The fluid within your eye that nourishes and fills the front and back chambers.

Aromatherapy Aromatherapy is an alternative therapy that is purported to enhance your well being through scent. The program includes wrapping your body in warm sheets saturated with scented oils. Then you are covered with a thermal blanket, as if you were in a cocoon. The manufacturers of these products claim benefits such as reduced swelling, pain reduction, and inhibited bacteria growth.

Arousal A.K.A. activation level.

Arrhythmia An abnormal heart rhythm. This is usually caused by a problem with your heart's electrical system.

Arteriosclerosis A.K.A. hardening of the arteries It refers to the fact that your arteries may become hard and brittle through the deposition of calcium on artery walls.

Artery A type of blood vessel that carries blood away from your heart.

Articular Processes These are two bony processes that are on the back part of each vertebra. They form your facet joints.

Association Focusing on the activity you are performing.

Asthma The wheeze of asthma is caused by contraction of the muscular walls of the small breathing tubes in your lungs. The narrowed air tube creates a turbulent air flow. This causes the wheezing or whistling when you breathe. Because the tubes into the lung are narrowed, less air can get in and this decreases the oxygen supply to your body. The pathological muscular contraction of your breathing tubes can be stimulated by a wide range of substances such as inhaled dust or pollen, and various foods.

Asthma and Exercise Carry your inhaler at all times during exercise. Keep your asthma under control so it doesn't interfere with your activity. If your doctor prescribed inhaled corticosteroids, use them according to your doctor's recommendations. Control your allergies. Visit your doctor regularly and follow his or her instructions about monitoring your condition. Be sure to report any concerns immediately.

Atherosclerosis Plaque and cholesterol build up along your artery walls. This causes a dangerous narrowing of your blood vessels.

Atherothrombotic Stroke This is a kind of stroke that happens after a large artery to your brain has already been narrowed by athlerosclerosis. It becomes completely blocked by the formation of a clot.

Athletic Shoes To find out if you need to replace tour shoes, place them on a table. Check for excessive wear. The back of your shoes should not slant inward. Shoes slanting inward may indicate overpronation, a condition in which your feet flatten and your ankles roll in. Worn spots on your shoes can also provide evidence of bone imbalances.

Atkins Diet A high-protein, low-carbohydrate, high-fat diet that has not been shown to be beneficial to long term weight loss.

Atrial Fibrillation A heart rhythm problem where your atria quivers ineffectually. This allows blood to sit idly and nonproductively, in your left atrium.

Atrium The upper chambers of your heart.

Atrophy If you quit using your muscles you lose them. Without stimulation, muscle atrophies.

Audience Arousal When someone is watching you perform a task, it increases your arousal.

Autonomic Nervous System (ANS) This is the part of your nervous system that controls involuntary, automatic, process. Examples include your heart beat and breathing.

Axon A part of the neuron that transmits a signal to a cell.

Basal Metabolic Rate (BMR) Your BMR is the amount of calories your body burns at rest. Your BMR includes sixty percent of your caloric burn from your functioning organs. Twenty five percent from your muscles. Ten percent from your bones. And five percent from fat.

Benign Prostatic Hyperplasia (BPH) An enlarged prostate that is not cancerous. It may interfere with urination.

Biceps These are the muscles on the front of your upper arm. They include your biceps brachii, brachialis, and brachioradialis.

Bilateral Transfer A theory stating that if you work a muscle group on one side of your body, it will enhance the muscle fibers on the other side of your body. For example, if you trained your right biceps muscle, your left biceps muscle would hypertrophy.

Bile This is the fluid that is secreted by your liver. Bile helps break down fats in your small intestine.

Bladder Infection A bladder infection (cystitis) is an inflammation of the wall and lining in your bladder. It may be caused by a bacterial infection or a mechanical abrasion from microcrystals of calcium phosphate in your urine. Symptoms of cystitis include frequent urination, dysuria (cloudy or bloody urine), with pain and tenderness in your lower abdomen. Your urine may be cloudy because it contains pus or blood and it may also have an unpleasant smell.

Blisters To prevent blisters, minimize friction. For the feet, this begins with your shoes. Shoes should fit comfortably the day that you buy them. There should be about a thumb's width between your longest toe and the end of your shoe. Narrow shoes cause blisters on your great toe and baby toe. A shallow toe box can cause blisters on the tops of your toes. Loose shoes can form blisters on the tips of your toes.

Body Mass Index The average body mass index score is 25. BMI stands for your weight in kilograms divided by your height in meters squared.

Body Fat Percentage Percent body fat is the ratio of fat to the rest of you (ie. muscle, bone, etc.). Men can reach as low as three percent fat. Women twelve percent. These are extremes. A reasonable goal for men to strive for might be ten to fifteen percent fat. Women fifteen to twenty percent.

Body Fat Storage Women have more subcutaneous body fat than men. But as both men and women age, body fat storage is more internal.

BodyPump The BodyPump class is designed to work your entire body using barbells with adjustable weights. The instructor cranks up the music, and leads you through a warm-up. Then a series of specifically choreographed moves, including squats, presses, lifts and curls are performed. You use light to moderate weights with high repetitions. The bar is three pounds with the option of adding additional weight.

Bolus A softened mass of chewed food. It ends up traveling down your esophagus into your stomach.

Bonk A.K.A. hitting the wall. A slang term used in endurance event where you run out of glycogen in your muscles and you cannot take another step or pedal stroke.

Boxaerobics An aerobic-anaerobic exercise program using punches, footwork, and blocks performed to the beat of lively music.

Bradykinesia "Brady" means slow. And "kinese" means movement. Slow movement.

Brain Stem This is the part of your brain that controls your breathing, heart rate, and other vital functions.

Breathing During Exercise You could virtually hold your breath while lifting weights, sprinting to your mailbox, or serving a tennis ball. But don't try it. Exhale with exertion and you will perform better, without blowing a gasket.

Broca's Area This part of your brain is located in your frontal left hemispheric lobe. It is responsible for your speech.

Bronchitis Bronchitis is the technical term for inflamed airways. Bronchitis can last from a few days to a few weeks. It normally occurs after a cold or flu. When bronchitis lasts for more than a few weeks, or strikes at least once a year, it is considered chronic. Bronchitis is rampant among smokers and people with lung disease.

Burn Fat You burn fat all day long. And all night too. But to burn fat most efficiently, a comfortable but challenging pace is your best steady-state speed to burn fat. It is not necessary to be in an "aerobic training zone" to burn fat. You burn fat all of the time. Even in your sleep. The more fit you are, the more aerobic enzymes you have, and the more fat you burn.

Bursitis A bursa is a pocket of connective tissue that sits next to a joint. It is lined by a smooth inner surface to help your muscles and tendons glide over nearby bones. Bursitis is inflammation of your bursa. It becomes painful, tender, and stiff. In some cases there is swelling and redness. Bursitis involving the shoulder, elbow, hip, and knee are the most common.

Caffeine We know that caffeine helps you to mobilize free fatty acids for your endurance events. And recent research also demonstrates that caffeine improves motor unit recruitment in trained weight lifters to increase the amount of weight they can hoist. Caffeine is found in coffee, tea, cola and chocolate. Although caffeine seems harmless, it can be highly addictive. More than a few cups of caffeine-containing beverages per day can cause fertility problems, ulcers, raise blood pressure, cause tachyarrhythmia (an abnormally increased heart rhythm), increased cholesterol, and trigger panic attacks.

Calcium Channel Blocker These are drugs that dilate your coronary arteries. They are used for reducing blood pressure in hypertensive patients.

Caloric Expenditure You can increase your total caloric expenditure by lifting weights, doing aerobics, eating small, frequent meals, and increasing your total activity throughout the day.

Calorie Some consider calories the enemy. Fat calories, in particular. You can get fat on too many fat, protein, or carbohydrate calories. But you need calories for growth, repair, and energy.

Cancer An abnormal growth or tumor in which cells multiply uncontrollably. Cancer can invade and spread to other parts of the body.

Capillary A vessel that transfers blood between your smallest arteries and your smallest veins.

Carb Loading Previously, athletes stopped eating carbohydrates five days before their event. They became grouchy and cantankerous. Then, in order to load their muscle glycogen stores, they ate all of the breads and pastas in sight. Recent studies suggest the carbohydrate depletion stage is unnecessary. Instead, athletes should taper their training and increase their carbohydrates as their event approaches. This loads glycogen stores without creating needless irritability.

Carbohydrates Carbohydrates (carbos) are not the enemy. Some of the latest fad diets claim that carbos make you fat. Carbohydrates include God-given potatoes, rice, beans, peas, corn, fruits, and grains. Processed carbohydrates are more calorically dense. These include pasta, bagels, and cereals. Carbos supply your muscles with energy to complete your workout.

Cardiac Output The amount of blood that your heart can pump in one minute.

Cardio vs Strength Training Which Shoud You Do First? Do your strength training first. This way, you can re-cycle that lactic acid from your weight-work to be used for energy during your cardio workout.

Cardio-Kickboxing An aerobic-anaerobic exercise program using punches, kicks, strikes, and blocks. Music is your motivation and an instructor teaches you your martial arts techniques practiced to the beat of music.

Cardiovascular This involves your heart, lungs, and blood vessels.

Carotid Arteries Blood vessels located on either sides of your neck. They supply blood to your brain.

Carpal Bones A.K.A. bones in your wrist.

Cartilage Replacement Healthy cartilage is taken from your knee. It's sent to Massachusetts where the cells are grown in a test tube. A month later, millions of cells are returned and injected back into your knee. Two hundred operations have been performed so far. The success rate has been ninety percent.

Cataract A clouding of the lens of your eye.

Catheter A hollow, flexible tube that is used to add or remove fluid from your body.

Celiac Disease Malabsorption of nutrients because of a sensitivity to gluten. Gluten is a protein found in wheat, rye, and barley. Symptoms include diarrhea, weight loss, and malnutrition.

Cerebellum This is the part of your brain that coordinates your movements.

Cerebral Cortex This is the part of your brain that is involved in thought, language, and memory.

Cerebrovascular Accident (CVA) A.K.A. stroke.

Chiropractor A practitioner who treats disease by manipulation of the spine and other body structures.

Cholesterol A fatlike substance, produced by your liver. Cholesterol is in all animal food sources. It is an essential component of body cells. It is a wax-like in appearance. If your total cholesterol is greater than 200 ml/dl, find out from your doctor your ratio of LDL to HDL. If your HDL is high, better than a 4:1 ratio, you're doing fine.

Chylomicron An extremely low-density lipoprotein. It transports triglycerides from your intestine to the fat cells in your body.

Chyme An almost liquid mass of partially digested food in your stomach and intestine.

Circuit Training Circuit training is a way to get two workouts for the price of one. If you do not have time for both aerobics and weight training, combine them with circuit training. Move from one exercise machine to the next, performing ten repetitions on each. Do not rest between exercises. The good news is, you will be huffing and puffing and your muscles will be pumped, all within the same workout. The bad news is, it would be more beneficial to separate your aerobics and strength training workouts to receive maximum benefit from both.

Cold Therapy The sooner you deal with swelling after an injury the better. Apply a cold compress directly to the injury immediately. Cold shrinks blood vessels, which reduces bleeding. This helps to prevent swelling. Cold also relieves pain and keeps your muscles from going into spasm.

Collagen A protein that provides your skin and other tissues form and tone.

Colon Your large intestine. It extends from your ileum to your rectum. It is divided into your ascending, transverse, descending, and sigmoid colon.

Compound Set Performing two or more exercises for the same muscle group.

Compression Fracture This is when one of your bones collapses. It happens most often in your vertebra.

Computerized Tomography (CT) This is a way for doctors to visualize what's going on in your body. X-rays are taken from many different angles. These pictures are fed into a computer to generate cross-sectional images of your body.

Concussion Receiving a blow to your head once in a contest is enough. The "second impact syndrome" happens when there are two consecutive impacts to your head without time for the first concussion to heal. The second impact can cause a coma or fatal brain swelling although the two individual hits seemed to be mild.

Cones These are cells in your retina. They are sensitive to color and light. Cones are most active during daylight. They provide you with sharp vision.

Conjunctiva This is your mucous membrane that lines your eyelid.

Contraction The cross-bridging of actin and myosin and the pulling together of these fibers to cause a muscle contraction.

Controlability Your ability to control the mental picture you have created in an attempt to improve your performance.

Cornea Your cornea is a curved, transparent tissue that is in the front part of your eye.

Coronary Arteries These are the arteries that supply your heart with blood.

Coronary Artery Disease (CAD) CAD is a narrowing or blockage of the arteries that supply blood to your heart muscle. Risk factors for CAD include cigarette smoking, elevated blood cholesterol, high blood pressure, and physical inactivity. Low levels of high-density lipoprotein cholesterol a.k.a. the "good cholesterol" also increases your risk.

Corpus Callosum This is a large bundle of nerve fibers linking your left and right cerebral hemispheres in your brain.

Creatine The only supplement in the last few years that has been shown to increase strength and size for bodybuilding athletes.

Cross-Training In cross-training, two or more types of exercise are performed in a single workout, or used alternately in successive workouts. A distance cyclist may run twice a week, perform daily stretching, and lift weights occasionally.

Crunches vs Walking To remove body fat, burn calories. The abdominal muscle group is relatively small, and the number of calories expended during crunches is minimal. Twenty minutes of walking will expend more calories than a couple of hundred crunches.

Cryotherapy This is where cold or freezing temperatures are used to treat disease.

Crystalline Lens This is a transparent body directly behind your iris. It focuses light onto your retina.

Dandruff Dandruff is sometimes associated with oily hair. A cause may be a yeast infection of your scalp. Hormonal and seasonal changes can also make dandruff worse. And sometimes dandruff may be the result of a dry scalp.

Definition in Your Muscle Most people think the way to lose the fat between your skin and muscle is to lift light weights and perform lots of repetitions. But muscular definition is a function of your eating, aerobics, and full body resistance training program. You may do hundreds of repetitions of crunches, but if a layer of fat surrounds your abdominals (abs), you will never see your "six pack."

Degenerative Spondylolisthesis This is where your facet joints gradually erode from wear and tear.

Dehydration Prevent dehydration by taking in water and electrolytes. Be sure you are getting enough potassium which is inside your muscle fibers, and calcium which is outside.

Deltoid A.K.A. shoulder. These muscles include your anterior deltoid, medial deltoid, and posterior deltoid.

Dermabrasion Using sandpaper or wire brushes to surgically remove skin blemishes or tatoos.

Dermatitis Dermatitis is a superficial inflammation of your skin. Contact dermatitis may be relieved by discontinuing use of industrial solvents, dyes, nickel, and other metals, and leather tanning chemicals.

Determining Percent Body Fat Under water weighing, electrical impedance, and calipers are three of the most reliable methods used to determine percent body fat.

Diabetes Mellitus A.K.A. Type II Diabetes This is considered adult onset. It is a disorder in which your blood glucose levels are elevated. The reason your blood sugar is high, is that insulin has a hard time dragging the sugar from your blood into your cells.

Diaphragm This is a flat layer of muscle that separates your chest from your abdomen. Your diaphragm helps you to breath. Breathing from your diaphragm helps you to relax.

Diastole Consider diastole the rest period between contractions of your heart. It is the bottom number of your blood pressure ratio (eg. 120/80).

Digestive Tract This is all of the organs that your food sees when it travels from your mouth to your anus.

Digital Rectal Examination (DRE) This is the dreaded gloved finger into the rectum test. Your doctor is checking out the size and texture of your prostate to decide if there are abnormalities.

Dihydrotestosterone (DHT) This is a biologically active form of testosterone. The bad news is that it stimulates prostate growth.

Diskectomy This is the surgical removal of all or part of one of your intervertebral disks.

Diskitis "Itis" means inflammation, so disk-itis refers to inflammation of your intervertebral disk.

Dissociation Keeping your mind on something else, rather than thinking about the activity you are doing.

Diverticula These are finger-shaped pouches in your colon that sometimes develop as you age.

Dopamine This is a neurotransmitter that helps you to move comfortably and smoothly.

Dry Hydro-Therapy Flotation Dry hydro-therapy flotation delivers power jets of heat to you while you are lying on a mattress. The water jets are designed to apply pressure to trigger points on muscles on your back, supposedly reducing pain, stimulating your nervous system, and reducing muscle spasms.

Duodenitis This is inflammation of your duodenum.

Duodenum This is the first section of your small intestine. It goes from your stomach to your jejunum.

Duration The duration of your workout session.

Dynamic Stretching Using your own muscle power to stretch your limbs through a range of motion.

Dyskinesia This malady refers to excessive and uncontrollable movements.

Dyspepsia Dyspepsia is similar to indigestion. It is characterized by upper abdominal pain following meals. Dyspepsia may be accompanied by bloating, nausea, vomiting, a sense of fullness, and general discomfort.

Dysphagia This is having difficulty in swallowing.

Eating After Exercise The carbohydrate window of opportunity is a fifteen minute period after a workout when your muscles are most receptive to take in recovery nutrients. Simple carbohydrates will do. Exercise provides a greater of volume of blood to your muscles. Your blood carries carbohydrates that were absorbed from the stomach. This causes maximum nutrient reabsorption into your muscles providing a more rapid recovery from exercise.

Echocardiography Doctors use echocardiography to provide them with a visualization of the heart. It uses ultrasound.

Ectomorph There are three distinct body types, and a variety of in-betweens. Ectomorphs are thin and small boned. They have a hard time putting on weight. Kate Moss is an example of an ectomorph.

Electrocardiogram (ECG) These are those wavy lines you see on the E.R. crash cart. ECG's record electrical activity within your heart.

Electromyography (EMG) This diagnostic procedure measures the electrical activity in your muscles.

Elliptical Machines One of the hottest items in gyms. You burn one and one half more calories moving backwards on an elliptical machine than forwards because you must use your stabilizer muscles in a different motor unit pattern.

Embolism A blood clot, or clump of material called an embolus blocks arterial blood flow and causes an embolism.

Encephalitis Inflammation of your brain.

Endomorph Endomorphs are big-boned, pear-shaped, and always seem to be on a diet. Most of us are on a continuum between body types. There are ecto-mesomorphs, ecto-endomorphs, and meso-endomorphs.

Endorphins A.K.A. the "runners high". Endorphins are a natural morphine-like substances produced in your body in response to pain, exercise, or the pain of exercise.

Endoscopy A doctor inserts a flexible tube down your throat to see your upper gastrointestinal tract.

Energy Bars Energy bars are tasty and convenient. But four researchers recently found that a bagel gives the same exercise performance benefits as an energy bar.

Enteric Nervous System (ENS) A complex network of nerves in your stomach wall that communicates with your brain.

Epinephrine A.K.A. adrenaline. A chemical that can act as a neurotransmitter or a hormone. It constricts your blood vessels and increases your heart rate.

Epithelium An outer layer of cells that line your stomach or skin.

Erector Spinae A long muscle mass that extends down your back. These muscles attach from your pelvis, to the bony processes of your vertebrae, and to your rib cage, and upper parts of your spine.

Esophagitis Inflammation of your esophagus.

Esophagus A.K.A. gullet. It is a tubular passageway from your pharynx to your stomach.

Estrogen A female sex hormone. But men have it too, at very low levels.

Estrogen-Replacement Therapy (ERT) As some women age, they decide to replace their declining hormones using ERT. They take estrogen to help prevent osteoporosis.

Exercise Stress Test A test used to determine your heart's response to exercise. It is usually administered in a hospital setting. While you are walking on a treadmill, an electrocardiogram measures how your heart handles the stress of exercise.

Exercise Regular vigorous exercise increases your need for calories and nutrients. Exercise improves your elimination and metabolism, which means you need to eat regularly. Physical exercise is also a stressor that may increase free-radical formation.

Extensor and Flexor Muscles A.K.A. forearm muscles.

External Obliques Your external obliques are your visible (if there is not a layer of fat covering them) "hands in your front pocket muscles." These muscles help you pull and twist, or reach across your body as you lean forward.

Facet Joints These are the tops and bottoms of your vertebra joints. The facets are located on the back side of each vertebra. They connect to the one above it, and the one below it.

Fast Twitch Muscle A.K.A. Type II b muscle fibers are white and powerful. They contract more quickly and forcefully than slow twitch, Type I, red fibers.

Fast Twitch/Slow Twitch Fibers What matters most is the load, not the speed of movement. Try this—lift up a two hundred pound weight. You wouldn't be able to lift it very fast (unless you are Hulk Hogan), but you would still be using fast twitch muscle fibers.

Fat Cells You developed your fat cells during the 3rd trimester in your mother's womb (so blame it on your mom), your first year of life (that's her fault again), and during puberty. It is also theorized you can add fat cells during pregnancy, and during explosive weight gain in adulthood.

Fat Loss You cannot "lose" fat cells, unless you undergo liposuction. But you may decrease the fat within each of your cells with proper diet and exercise.

Fatty Acids These are the primary building blocks of fats (lipids).

Female Athletic Triad Female athletic triad is a newly recognized link between eating disorders, amenorrhea (lack of menstruation), and osteoporosis. The combination of disordered eating and amenorrhea cause weakness in bones leading to osteoporosis.

Festinating Gait You may have noticed your grandfather shuffling with small steps while hunched forward. It is as though he was chasing his center of gravity.

Fiber Type Your parents are responsible for your fiber type. You will never be as fast as Donovan Bailey if you were not blessed with a preponderance of white fast twitch fibers.

Fiber A.K.A. roughage. Fiber is found in plant foods as an indigestible form of carbohydrate. Fiber provides plants with their "upright" structure. Soluble fibers dissolve in water. Insoluble fibers do not. Most plants contain both types.

Fibrous Plaque An advanced form of atherosclerotic plaque. It forms in response to an injury on the inside lining of your blood vessel.

Finasteride It was first designed as a drug to treat benign prostate hyperplasia (BPH). It shrinks the prostate by interfering with the action of 5-alpha reductase, an enzyme that converts testosterone to dihydrotestosterone. Dihydrotestosterone stimulates prostate growth. Recently some "genius" discovered that finasteride grows hair. It's new, expensive name is Propecia.

Fine Motor Task A small muscle movement such as putting in golf.

Floaters You may have seen these flit across the horizon. They are clusters of protein or cells that drift through the vitreous humor in your eye and appear as black specks across your visual field. If you see these regularly, call your opthamologist. Seeing floaters may be an early warning sign of retinal problems.

Flow A mindful experience where there is no ego, competition, anxiety, or boredom. An alpha state that allows you to perform your activity on automatic.

Fluoride It may be found in your tap water. Fluoride is a compound that can increase bone density, and is a possible treatment for osteoporosis.

Foot Pain When you walk, you are slamming about one-times your body weight on each foot fall. In running, it's two-and-a-half to three times your body weight pounding through your feet, knees and back. Ignoring pain can lead to irreversible damage to your back, feet, or knees.

Free Fragment A free fragment is not something you want, even if it is free. A free fragment is a displaced portion of your intervertebral disk. It detaches from the central portion of the disk.

Free Radicals Molecules in your body have two electrons in their outer shell. A molecule with one electron in its outer shell is called a free radical. It is searching for a free electron. While it is trying to bind with another electron to complete itself, it can damage your organs and tissue. Free radicals occur when oxygen in the bloodstream combines with polluted air, cigarette smoke, food additives, and re-heated cooking oil. Free radical production and damage is increased by exercise—especially running and other aerobics because there is more oxygen in your bloodstream.

Free Weights Free weights allow you to follow the natural line of pull of your muscles. Free weights also require you to use stabilizer muscles to balance the weight. Free weights also let you pre-stretch your muscles to their optimum 1.2 times their resting length just before you make your lift. These are some of the reasons that professional bodybuilders seem to prefer free weights over machines.

Frequency How many times a week you work out.

Frontal Lobe Remember all those movies that threatened a "frontal lobotomy?" Actually, your frontal lobe is one of four major subdivisions of the two hemispheres of your brain. It is important for helping you control your movement.

Fructose Some folks think because fructose is fat-free it is calorie-free. It is not. Fructose is a simple sugar found in corn syrup, honey, and many fruits.

Gall Bladder Disease Gall bladder disease is characterized by severe pain that becomes localized in the upper right quadrant of your abdomen, radiating to your right lower scapula (shoulder blade). Nausea and vomiting are common. Diet is important, as any fats consumed will precipitate the pain.

Gastritis A.K.A. inflammation of the stomach.

Gastrocnemius A.K.A. calf muscle. The long, sleek muscle on your lower leg.

Gastroesophageal Reflux Disease (GERD) A.K.A. heartburn, GERD is a condition in which food and acid flow back into your esophagus from your stomach. The acid may damage your esophagus.

Gastrointestinal (GI) Tract A.K.A. digestive tract.

Glomeruli These are the tiny structures within your kidneys that filter waste products from your blood.

Glucose Intolerance This means that you have trouble getting sugar from your bloodstream into your cells.

Glucose A.K.A. sugar. Your body's main source of energy. Glucose comes mainly from the digestion of carbohydrates.

Gluteal Muscles A.K.A. butt. This is the largest muscle group in your body.

Golf Injury Prevention and Health Lift your clubs out of your car with your legs not your back. Arrive at the course ten minutes early and do some stretching exercises for your back, shoulders, and legs. Walk the course instead of riding. Begin your practice sessions with a nine iron and work your way to a five iron. On cool days, wear layers of clothes. If you feel pain during your swing, stop immediately. Check with a golf pro and physical therapist for strengthening and stretching exercises to improve the mechanics of your swing.

Golf Strength Training A few old-fogey golfers believe the myth that muscle-strengthening exercises such as weight training can hurt their golf game. Golf is a sport. And sportsmen train with weights. Check out pro golfers. They understand that a stronger and more flexible body will help keep their fitness levels up and their scores down.

Golgi Tendon Organ When you stretch a muscle, you can activate your golgi tendon organ. Your golgi tendon organ relaxes the muscle so that it will not become injured. For example if you are trying to lift a weight off of the floor and it is too heavy for your muscles to support, your golgi tendon organ will cause your muscles to relax and you will drop the weight.

Gout An attack of acute gouty arthritis is caused by the formation of needlelike, crystals of uric acid. Uric acid is a metabolite of your urine. When extreme, large deposits of uric acid surrounds joints, gout occurs acutely as intermittent attacks of joint pain. There is swelling, redness, and warmth. In some individuals, it is a progressive, crippling, chronic disease that also damages the kidneys.

Grains Grains are the seeds or fruits of cereal grasses. The unprocessed kernels are several layers surrounding a core. An outer, inedible layer called the hull, protects the entire seed. A layer of bran, made up of indigestible fiber and containing iron, thiamin, niacin, riboflavin, and some protein is inside the hull. The germ is surrounded by the endosperm, a layer of starch inside a protein matrix. In the core is the germ, which contains unsaturated fat, protein, iron, niacin, thiamin, and riboflavin.

Gross Motor Task A large muscle movement such as pushing a refrigerator.

Gullet A.K.A. esophagus.

Half-Bench Squats Don't use a bench to rest on for half squats. Your stabilizer muscles in your spine relax forcing you to lose stability.

Hamstrings The muscles on the back of your upper leg. It is made up of your semitendinosis, semimembranosis, and biceps femoris.

HDL Cholesterol There are two types of cholesterol. Well, actually three. High density lipoproteins (HDL)—the good cholesterol, Low Density Lipoproteins (LDL)—the bad cholesterol, and Very Low Density Lipoproteins(VLDL)—also bad guys.

Heart Failure This is where your heart loses its ability to efficiently pump blood throughout body.

Heart Rate Training Monitoring your heart rate while you perform anaerobic and aerobic training to reach certain heart rate levels.

Heartburn Digestive juices usually follow gravity; they go down, not up. But if digestive juices go up, there is a problem. It's called heartburn. Your throat feels on fire and there may be pressure under your ribs. It's not very pleasant, but it is common.

Helicobacter Pylori (H. Pylori) A spiral bacterium found at the surface of the stomach epithelium has recently been shown to be a major cause of gastritis and peptic ulcer disease.

Hematuria Hematuria or blood in your urine may be associated with a wide range of conditions. The bleeding will occur at a site of physical trauma, such as a stone cutting the tissue or bleeding from an infection. Your urine becomes red or brown in color. If the amount of blood is small it might not be noticed, but it can be detected by a number of simple tests.

Hemorrhagic Stroke A type of stroke that occurs when a blood vessel ruptures. This cuts off the supply of oxygen and nutrition to parts of your brain. High blood pressure is the main cause of such strokes.

Hemorrhoids Hemorrhoids are cushions of tissue that line your lower rectum. They serve to produce complete closure of your anal canal. Symptoms of hemorrhoids are bleeding, protrusion, and pain.

Heparin An anticoagulant drug that inhibits blood from clotting. It interferes with coagulation factors. Heparin is usually administered in the hospital either by an injection or an intravenous line.

Herniated Disk Very painful. A herniated disk is a displacement of some portion of one of your spinal disks out of its normal location.

Hiatal Hernia Part of your stomach protrudes into your chest through an opening in your diaphragm.

High Density Lipoprotein (HDL) A.K.A. good cholesterol. HDL is a lipoprotein that protects the arteries by transporting cholesterol from body cells to the liver for elimination.

Hippocampus A part of your brain's limbic system that is involved in learning, memory, and emotion.

Histamine A chemical present in specific cells throughout your body. It is a mediator of allergic reactions.

Holter Monitor A portable device that you wear continuously to measure electrical activity of your heart.

Home Workout Machines A machine can be well-made but still feel funny. Try the machine in the store. How do your lower back, joints, and muscles feel? Your seat should be comfortable during long exercise sessions. Bars or pull-handles should be padded and feel okay even after several minutes. How hard are the control knobs to adjust? Is the machine too noisy for your home?

Hormone Therapy Using drugs to keep male hormones such as testosterone from stimulating the growth of prostate cancer cells.

Hormone-Replacement Therapy (HRT) HRT augments a woman's depleted hormones after she reaches menopause. HRT is a combination of estrogen and progesterone. The purpose of HRT is to reduce osteoporosis risk.

Hormones These are chemical released from glands into your bloodstream. They affect organs or tissues elsewhere in your body.

Humerus Upper arm bone.

Hydrogen Breath Test A diagnostic test for carbohydrate malabsorption. The test measures the amount of hydrogen in your exhaled breath.

Hydrogenation Check the ingredients on the wrapper of your candy bar for the word "hydrogenated." Hydrogenation means the addition of hydrogen to a substance. It makes unsaturated oils and soft fats hard.

Hyperglycemia This is a measure of high levels of glucose (sugar) in your blood.

Hyperlipidemia A measure of high levels of blood fats (lipids).

Hypertension A.K.A. high blood pressure. High blood pressure is a major risk factor for stroke. Hypertension causes excess stress on the walls of your blood vessels and damages their delicate inner lining.

Hyperthyroidism Overactivity of your thyroid gland is called hyperthyroidism.

Hypertrophy A.K.A. muscle growth.

Hypothyroidism Hypothyroidism is an under activity of your thyroid. It results in too little production of thyroid hormone. Although hypothyroidism may be caused by a variety of diseases that affect the hypothalamus and pituitary gland, this condition is usually due to disorders of the thyroid gland itself.

Ice-Heat Therapy Ice is your first line of defense against injury. Heat is the second component. Heat will soften your tightened muscle and cause blood to flush the area. This enhances oxygen and nutrient delivery to your deprived and tightened muscle.

Idiopathic Think of the word "idiot" on this one. Doctors often say it is idiopathic which means without a known cause.

Ileum This is the section of your small intestine between your jejunum and the beginning of your large intestine.

Iliopsoas Muscles A.K.A. hip flexor. These two muscles are located on each side of your lumbar vertebrae and are attached to them. They are on the inside of your pelvis and are connected to your thigh bones. They help you to lift your knee.

Imagery A psychological strategy designed to help you improve your physical performance.

Infarction The death of cells due to lack of blood. Infarction is usually preceded by lack of oxygen (ischemia).

Inflammation Inflammation is a process that occurs in response to a range of traumas from sunburn and wounds, to infection and auto-immune conditions. Whatever the cause, the process leads to warmth, redness, swelling, and pain.

Insomnia Insomnia, or sleeplessness may be caused by a variety of triggers. The key to successful treatment of insomnia is to find the cause and deal with it. Whether the cause is emotional, physical, or environmental (a snoring spouse), seek out the cause of your insomnia to uncover the cure.

Instructor Motivation A group exercise leader can increase your motivation to burn an additional two calories per minute.

Insulin A hormone produced by your pancreas. Insulin helps blood glucose (sugar) get into your cells.

Insulin-Dependent Diabetes A.K.A. Type I or Juvenile onset diabetes. It usually appears before age thirty-five. People with diabetes need insulin injections because their bodies have stopped producing it.

Intensity How hard you work out.

Internal Obliques Your internal obliques are beneath your external obliques. They form the shape of a roof top. Your right internal oblique turns you to the right. And your left internal oblique turns you to the left.

Intervertebral Disk A.K.A. the shock absorbers of your spine. They are small, energy-absorbing, sponge-like cushions located between the vertebrae of your spine.

Iris Your iris shows whether you have brown, green, or blue eyes. It is the colored ring in front of your lens that controls the size of the pupil and how much light enters gets in.

Irritable Bowel Syndrome There are a variety symptoms that can occur in this condition. They may include abdominal distress, erratic frequency of bowel movements, bloating, flatulence, and variability in stool consistency.

Ischemia A dangerous decrease in the supply of blood to tissue. Ischemia is usually caused by atherosclerotic narrowing of the vessel.

Isokinetic A cybex type of weight machine that uses a constant resistance as it takes your muscle through a full range of motion. These machines may be used for training, rehabilitation, and testing.

Isometric Pushing against an immovable object. Your muscles contract but there is no movement.

Isotonic Free weight training. Hoisting weights where the resistance remains the same, but gravity makes the exercises easier or more difficult through different ranges of motion.

Jejunum This is the section of your small intestine between your duodenum and ileum.

Kid's Weight Training Running and jumping has the same effect on bones as weight training and neither seem to cause premature closure of epiphyseal bone plates.

Kyphosis This is commonly called dowager's hump and refers to an abnormal front-to-back curvature of your mid-to-upper spine. It can be the result of compression fractures of your vertebrae.

Lactase An enzyme in your intestine that breaks down lactose.

Lactose Intolerance The inability of your body to absorb lactose. Drinking milk products causes gastrointestinal distress.

Lactose A sugar. It is found in milk and dairy products.

Lamina One of the two thin, platelike parts of each of your vertebra. They join in the midline and form the base of the spinous process of that vertebra.

Laminectomy An operation in which all of, or a portion of one or both laminae is removed. The purpose of a laminectomy is to gain access to the spinal canal, or to decompress the spinal cord and nerve roots.

Lattisimus Dorsi The long, wide muscle of your back. When it is developed, it takes the shape of wings.

LDL Low-Density Lipoprotein. A.K.A. bad cholesterol. A type of cholesterol that is implicated in the development of atherosclerotic plaques.

Left Ventricular Hypertrophy A thickening of the wall of the left ventricle of your heart. Heavy weight training has been implicated in producing left ventricular hypertrophy.

Ligament Connects bone to bone.

Limbic System The part of your brain that contains your amygdala, hippocampus, and the basal ganglia. It affects emotion, memory, and certain aspects of movement.

Lipase An enzyme that is secreted by your pancreas that helps digest fats.

Lipids A.K.A. Fats, oils, and waxes. They serve as building blocks for cells or as energy sources for the body.

Lipoprotein Analysis When you get your cholesterol tested, always ask for a lipoprotein analysis. This laboratory test determines the relative levels of HDL and LDL in your blood.

Lipoproteins These are protein covered fat particles. They enable cholesterol and triglycerides to move easily through your blood.

Liposuction Liposuction is the surgical removal of fat cells and their contents. It is not a pretty procedure. Try an eating and exercise program first. After all else fails, and you cannot lose your saddlebags, and you have lost fat everywhere else, and you are obsessed about pinching no more than an inch, you may be a candidate for liposuction. If you undergo liposuction to remove fat from your hips, but you continue to eat with reckless abandon, your fat stores will balloon somewhere else.

Liver Not very tasty, but it is your body's largest internal organ. It secretes bile and is part of many metabolic functions.

Low Back Pain Females have a slightly greater incidence of low back pain than men because their pelvis' tilt forward causing a more pronounced lordotic curve. Exercise helps to prevent low back pain by promoting calcium formation and increasing bone nutrition.

Low Carbohydrate Diets Carbohydrate-bashing diets claim that carbos are bad because they increase blood sugar and cause insulin to be released. Supposedly this is a bad thing. Proponents of these diets say insulin causes high-carbohydrate foods to be stored as fat rather than used for energy. This is just not true!

Lumbar Spine A.K.A. lower back. This is the five lower vertebrae of your spine.

Lung Problems Training For maximum benefits, walk or pedal at a rate that raises your heart rate to sixty percent to eighty percent of its maximum, for thirty minutes, three days a week. It may take days, weeks, or months to reach that goal, or you may never get there at all. But that doesn't matter. Your goal is to improve your ability to exercise. Any improvement is great. Lung patients may make tremendous gains. In six weeks, you might see a seventy percent to eighty percent improvement over your initial workouts.

Lunges Lunges are great for training your glutes and thighs.

Lupus Systemic Lupus Erythematosus (S.L.E.) is a multi-symptom, multi-organ connective tissue disease that primarily affects women of child-bearing age. SLE tends to run in families. While no specific cause has been identified, there are thought to be many different triggers.

Lymph Nodes These are glands that are part of your immune system. They help your body fight off disease.

Lymphoma A malignant tumor of the lymph tissue.

Magnetic Resonance Imaging (MRI) Doctors use this computerized imaging strategy to see different tissues in your body in a variety of planes. Radio waves generated in a strong magnetic field are used to provide information about the hydrogen atoms in different tissues within your body

Malignant This refers to a tissue that is cancerous. It usually means the cancerous tumor will spread.

Massage Muscles typically tighten after exercise. The speed of recovery is directly related to the amount of blood that can enter the muscle to provide the necessary food and oxygen. Deep massage immediately after exercise encourages blood to enter a more relaxed muscle. Get a massage fifteen minutes after exercising, and several times during the rest of the day. Each session only needs to be forty-five to sixty seconds.

Mesomorph Mesomorphs have little problem gaining muscle. They have small waists and look like they workout all the time, even if they do not. Herschel Walker is a mesomorph.

Mind/Body Recovery Successful rehabilitation begins with learning about your injury. Know the extent of your injury, what your recovery time will be, and what you must do to recover. A recent cool study showed that just by thinking about doing a biceps curl, you actually produce muscular activity in your biceps.

Minerals Some athletes think they need doses of minerals to enhance their physical training. But studies show that, except for iron (particularly among female athletes), the mineral needs of highly trained athletes are similar to those of the general population. Furthermore, physical training does not inordinately deplete minerals.

Monounsaturated Fats (MUFAs) A.K.A. the "good" fats. Fatty acids, abundant in olive, peanut, sesame, and canola oils, in which one pair of hydrogen atoms in each molecule has been replaced by a double bond.

Motility This refers to the speed and capability of your digestive tract to propel its contents through your system.

Motor Unit A motor neuron and all of the muscle fibers it innervates.

Mucosa The inner lining of your stomach.

Muscle Cramp A muscle cramp is when your muscle contracts and shortens causing a sudden, severe pain. Muscle cramps are mostly caused by overexertion and dehydration. When you dehydrated, there is an electrolyte imbalance, and your muscles to cramp up. Electrolytes are minerals such as sodium, magnesium, calcium and potassium. An imbalance occurs when we have too much or too little of one or more electrolytes in our system. The main electrolytes affecting muscle cramping are potassium, sodium and calcium.

Muscle Metabolism You should eat enough calories to maintain your BMR. If not, your metabolism will slow, and you will store fat more efficiently.

Muscle/Fat Muscle does not turn into fat. Muscle and fat are two separate entities. If you lose muscle your metabolism slows. If you eat more calories than you burn, you gain fat.

Muscle Muscle is precious. Seventy-five percent of your muscle is water, twenty percent is protein, and five percent minerals. You have more than four hundred voluntary muscles in your body. Muscle makes up about half of your body weight. The more muscle you have the more calories your body burns. Muscle is metabolically active.

Muscle-Bound The colloquialism "muscle-bound" is a lack of flexibility due to tremendous amounts of muscle. I have yet to meet anyone with so much muscle that it "bound" him up. I have met folks who do not exercise, and have a restricted range of motion, however. If your reason for not lifting weights is you are afraid to become muscle-bound, find another excuse.

Myelography Doctors use this diagnostic technique to X-ray your spine. The doctor injects a contrast medium into the space within the sheath that surrounds your spinal cord. Your radiologist looks for herniated disks, tumors, and fractures.

Myofascial Release Myofascial release is using pressure from your arms and fingers to lengthen muscle and connective tissue. It is used in combination with physical therapy methods to relieve pain and stiffness.

Nerve paralysis There are three major types of nerve destruction that cause paralysis. Children may be born with an incomplete nervous system, such as spina bifida. An accident may occur that destroys part of the nervous system. Or a disease may destroy nervous tissue.

Neurologist A doctor trained to treat disorders of your brain and nervous system.

Neuron A nerve cell.

Neurotransmitter This is a chemical that is released by neurons at a synapse. It transmits information to other nerve cells.

Neutropenia A low count of white blood cells.

Non-Insulin-Dependent Diabetes A.K.A. adult onset diabetes. Often called Type II, it occurs mainly after age forty. Your body produces insulin, but not enough to meet your needs. In most cases it can be controlled by diet, exercise, and weight loss.

Norepinephrine This neurotransmitter constricts your blood vessels. It is released by your sympathetic nervous system.

Nucleus Pulposus This is the gel-like center of each of your intervertebral disks.

Obstructive Sleep Apnea (OSA) Your spouse may tell you that you stop breathing during sleep. OSA is characterized by heavy snoring and interrupted breathing during sleep.

Occipital Lobe This is one of the four major subdivisions of the two hemisphere of your brain. It is important for in visual perception.

Olecranon Process A.K.A. elbow.

Ophthalmologist A doctor who is a specialist in eye disease.

Optimum Level of Arousal Not too bored or too anxious. At a perfect energy level for the activity you are performing.

Orbit The bony socket that surround your eyeball.

Osgood-Schlatters Disease (OSD) OSD is an inflammation where the tendon from the kneecap attaches to the shin bone. Teens are particularly susceptible to these stresses because the bones are growing rapidly. Any activity can cause OSD, but it's common in jumping and cutting, like basketball, volleyball, soccer, figure skating, and gymnastics.

Osteoarthritis Osteoarthritis is, in a word, wear and tear on your joints. It is a degenerative joint disease that usually affects people over the age of forty-five. Or it can affect you if you have suffered joint injuries.

Osteoblast A bone-producing cell.

Osteoclast A bone-destroying cell.

Osteomyelitis Bone infection. Caused by fungi or bacteria.

Osteoporosis Osteoporosis is a thinning of your bones as you age. Your bones become more porous. Exercise is part of the treatment. As regular workouts build muscle, they also maintain and may even increase bone density. Older adults can strengthen their muscles and bones and improve their balance, thereby reducing their risk of falls and resulting fractures. For women, exercise works in combination with estrogen or other medications that increase bone density and strength. Exercise, medication, and proper diet fights osteoporosis more effectively together than any one treatment.

Overtraining The same motivation that you have to train hard and perform well can get you into trouble. Working too hard over a long period of time can cause overtraining. Overtraining hurts your performance and can cause sickness or injury. If you overtrain, you are out of balance. If your training program exceeds your rest time, you may be pushing your limits.

Pancreas A gland located behind your stomach. It secretes digestive enzymes, notably insulin.

Pancreatitis Inflammation of your pancreas.

Parasympathetic Nervous System One of the two branches of your autonomic nervous system. It helps to regulate digestion, circulation, voiding, and other bodily functions.

Parathyroid Hormone A hormone, made by four tiny pieces of tissue near your thyroid. It prevents your level of blood calcium from going too low.

Parietal Lobe One of the four major subdivision of the two hemispheres of your brain. It is important in sensory processes and language.

Passive Stretching Using a partner to take one of your limbs through a range of motion.

Patella A.K.A. kneecap.

Pectorals A.K.A. chest. These muscles include your pectoralis major and pectoralis minor.

Pepsin A name for several enzymes secreted by your stomach. Their job is to break down protein.

Percutaneous Diskectomy A doctor removes part of your intervertebral disk. A narrow probe is inserted through the skin and muscle of your back.

Peripheral Vision Side vision. This is what you can see outside of your direct line of vision.

Peristalsis Muscles in your intestine move in a wave-like fashion to propel food along your digestive tract.

Peritonitis Inflammation of the membrane lining your abdominal cavity.

Physiatrist A medical doctor who is trained as a rehabilitation specialist.

Phytochemicals Substances in fruits and vegetables that recently have been shown to fight cardiovascular disease and cancer.

Pilates Pilates(puh-la-tease) is named after Joseph Pilates who developed it in Germany in the 1920s. It was a favorite exercise for dancers who wanted to strengthen their muscles and soothe their aches and strains. Now it's the rage among those burned out on regular weight training. Proponents of Pilates suggest that it lengthens and strengthens muscle, while improving balance and posture.

Placebo Effect A.K.A. sugar pill. Your condition improved. But whatever helped you wasn't in the pill you were taking. From chromium picolinate to shark cartilage, people think more of supplements than they are worth. Folks swear to me the benefits of colloidal minerals and magnets. Benjamin Franklin painted blocks of wood black. People thought they were magnets. They slept with these blocks of wood because they believed magnets cured arthritis. Miraculously, they were healed. The blocks of wood worked!

Plaque A fatty buildup of cholesterol, calcium, and other substances inside your blood vessels.

Platelets Tiny, colorless disks in your blood that help your clotting mechanism.

Plyometrics Makes use of your myotatic stretch reflex to pre-stretch your muscle prior to exploding through your designated range of motion.

Polyunsaturated Fats (PUFAs) A.K.A. the good fats. These are fatty acids found in soybean, corn, cottonseed, safflower, and sunflower oils. Two or more pairs of hydrogen atoms in each molecule have been replaced by double bonds.

Presbyopia A.K.A. farsightedness. This is the natural loss of your eye's ability to focus on close objects. It becomes prevalent in people over forty year old. But it can be corrected with reading glasses.

Process Bony projections that emanate from each of your vertebra

Prone A.K.A. lying on your tummy.

Proprioceptive Neuromuscular Facilitation (PNF) A type of stretching where you take your partners limb through a passive stretch. When your partner feels tension in the muscle, he/she presses against you for three seconds. Then he/she relaxes and you once again attempt to move your partners limb a little deeper into the stretch. The purpose of PNF is to activate your golgi tendon organ to relax your muscle and provide for a further stretch.

Proprioceptive Training A.K.A. balance training.

Prostate A walnut-shaped gland positioned at the base of the male bladder.

Prostatitis Prostatitis is an infection of the Prostate Gland. Symptoms include an aching pain in the area of the prostate. Pressure to the prostate gland is painful enough so that sitting may hurt. Other symptoms include trouble urinating, dribbling, and urinating often at night. Acute cases may be accompanied by fever.

Protein Protein is made up of chains of amino acids. Your body can make some, but not others. Protein is essential for building and maintaining muscles. Protein also repairs muscle damage that occurs during training. Protein also helps to make red blood cells, produce hormones, boost your immune system, and help keep hair, fingernails, and skin healthy.

Pseudoephedrine A decongestant drug.

Pursed-Lipped Breathing Used to slow your exhalation by forming your lips as if you were whistling.

Quadratus Lomborum Lower back muscles.

Quadriceps A.K.A. thigh muscles. A group of four muscles.

Reaction Time From the moment you think about starting your movement, until your muscles take action.

Reciprocal Inhibition When you contract a muscle group, the opposite muscle group (antagonist) automatically relaxes.

Rectum This is the final segment of your gastrointestinal tract. It is located between your sigmoid colon and anus.

Rectus Abdominis Your abdominals consist of several muscle groups. Your rectus abdominis is a long strap-like muscle extending from your lower-middle rib cage to your pubis. It lifts you into a sitting position each morning. It is your "six pack."

Regular Exercise Regular exercise can help control high blood pressure. A few sessions of moderate physical activity each week can reduce blood pressure significantly, and at the same time, lower your risk of stroke and heart attack. If your blood pressure is just mildly elevated, exercise, along with a healthy diet, and stress management, may be enough to bring it down. If you require medication, exercise will probably make it more effective, and possibly allow you to lower the dosages with your doctors recommendation.

Relaxed Concentration An alpha brain wave pattern where your mind and body are relaxed, but you are exquisitely focused on your task at hand.

Remodeling Your body's way of systematically removing old bone tissue and replacing it with new. This preserves the strength of your skeleton.

Rest-Pause Pausing at the bottom of each repetition of your set for just an instant to recruit more muscle fibers.

Retina The innermost layer of your eye. It converts light energy to electrical energy. It sends visual images to your brain through the connecting optic nerve.

Retinal Detachment A condition in which the retina separates from the choroid. Often seen in boxers.

Rheumatoid Arthritis Rheumatoid arthritis is an inflammatory autoimmune disease. It can strike folks aged thirty to forty, but most frequently attacks people in their fifties and sixties. Rheumatoid arthritis is more common in women. It is more serious than osteoarthritis because it can assault other tissues in your body, not just your joints.

Rheumatologist A doctor trained to diagnose and treat joints and other parts of the musculoskeletal system.

Rhomboids These are the muscles between your shoulder blades. These muscles help you to keep your shoulders back.

Rolfing The massage technique called rolfing was designed to fight the effects of gravity. Some folks with back and neck problems say it releases their tension and relieves their pain.

Rotator Cuff Muscles Supraspinatus, infraspinatus, teres minor, and subscapularis.

Rotator Cuff The rotator cuff is four muscles with a common tendon. Their function is to internally rotate (backhand in tennis) and externally rotate (throwing motion) your arm. Your rotator cuff is an important stabilizer of your shoulder during any throwing motion.

Rowing Machines Novice rowers glide on the forward, eccentric, movement so that there is too much rest to provide an excellent training effect.

Rubella A.K.A. German measles.

Salivary Gland This is where digestion begins. Your salivary gland is one of three pairs of glands that pour lubricating fluids into your mouth.

Sartorius The longest muscle in your body. It crosses both your hip and your knee.

Saturated Fats A.K.A. "bad" fats. These are fatty acids, abundant in red meat, lard, butter, hard cheeses, and some vegetable oils (palm, coconut, and cocoa butter) and partially hydrogenated oils. Each molecule carries the maximum amount of hydrogen atoms.

Scapulae A.K.A. shoulder blades.

Sciatica Pain along the course of your sciatic nerve. This can be from your buttock, down the back and side of your leg, and into your foot and toes. It is often because of a herniated disk.

Sclera A tough, protective coating of collagen and elastic tissue. This is the whites of your eyes.

Scoliosis An abnormal lateral "S" curvature of the spine.

Short Leg Syndrome Do you have any symptoms that are exaggerated by running, such as low back pain, hip, knee, ankle or foot pain? Do you repeatedly pull the same muscles even though you have given them sufficient time to heal? Do you get shin splints and sciatica (inflammation of the sciatic nerve that produces pain in the buttocks and down the back of the leg)? If so, these may be symptoms of having one leg significantly shorter than the other.

Small Intestine A section of your digestive system that includes your duodenum, jejunum, and ileum. It helps absorb nutrients for your body.

Soleus The muscle underneath your calf muscle. It adds volume to your lower leg. It is made up of predominantly slow twitch muscle fibers.

Soy Reduced risks of some diseases have been shown in populations that consume soy. Japanese and Chinese people have lower rates of heart disease and breast/prostate cancer than Americans. Soy may be a part of the explanation. Soy might also be of benefit to menopausal women.

Sphygmomanometer A device used to measure blood pressure.

Spinal Fusion Joining two or more vertebrae with a bone graft. This operation is performed in order to eliminate motion and relieve pain.

Spinal Stenosis A reduction in the size of your spinal canal. This may result in compression of your spinal cord or nerve roots.

Spinous Process These are the lever-like, backward projections from each of your vertebra. Muscles and ligaments attach to these.

Spondylolisthesis Forward displacement of one of your vertebra in relation to a vertebra immediately below.

Sprain Damage to a ligament.

Starting a Program Your body burns more calories sprinting than walking for the same time period. But begin easy. When you become more fit you can workout harder.

Static Stretching Holding your stretch at a point of tension.

Stepper Machines The speed that you step does not affect your caloric burn because the slower you go, the deeper you step.

Stomach The hollow, saclike organ of your digestive system. It lies between your esophagus and duodenum. Your stomach stores and grinds food. It secretes acid and digestive juices that break down proteins, and pushes chyme into the small intestine.

Strain Damage to a muscle or tendon.

Stress Stress is the response of your body to any demand. Just staying alive creates demands on your body, so you are always under stress. Even while you sleep, your body continues to function. Stress cannot be avoided nor should it be. Stress is linked to problems like high blood pressure and heart disease. It also exacerbates headaches, backaches, and digestive troubles. Stress can make your body aches more painful, your queasy stomach more upset, or worsen any of your symptoms, no matter what the original cause.

Stretch Reflex When you stretch a muscle too hard or too fast, it will contract to protect itself.

Stretching A combination of massage and stretching is the perfect medicine for tightened muscles after a workout. Use massage to relax your muscles. Now your muscle is prepared for recovery stretching. This keeps your muscles from tightening and shortens recovery time.

Stroke A stroke is caused by a disturbance of the blood supply to your brain. The blood vessels that normally supply blood to your brain can become blocked. This results in not enough blood getting to your brain. A stroke may be caused by raised blood pressure, hardening of the arteries, or a severe head injury. The functional impairment that occurs with a stroke depends on the area of the brain that is damaged.

Substrate Cycling Athletes adjust their voluminous training to their eating so that they can eat voraciously to make up for caloric loss, and workout again, and eat, and workout.

Superset Working antagonist muscle groups consecutively.

Super-Slow Training Performing a set of exercises where each repetition may last from four to ten seconds. The goal is to recruit more muscle fibers.

Supine A.K.A. lying on your back.

Supplements If you are going to use supplements, they should be used in addition to an eating and exercise program, not in replacement of. As long as supplement companies claims their products are foods, their advertising is virtually unregulated. Be careful.

Sympathetic Nervous System (SNS) One of two divisions of your autonomic nervous system. Your SNS prepares your body for action. Your blood pressure, heart and breathing rate increase to prepare for an emergency.

Synapse A tiny space between an axon terminal that fires off a chemical signal and the neuron that receives it.

Systolic Blood Pressure When you get your blood pressure taken, this is the number on top. It signifies the pressure in your arteries when your heart contracts.

Tarsal Bones A.K.A. bones in your ankle.

Temporal Lobe This is one of the four major subdivisions of the two hemispheres of your brain. Your temporal lobe is responsible for hearing, long-term memory, and behavior.

Tendinitis Tendons are strong, fibrous tissues that connect muscle to bone. When your tendon swells and becomes sore we call it tendinitis. There are several causes of tendinitis. One of the biggest is overuse of your muscles. Not stretching properly is another cause of tendinitis. Flexibility is important in preventing tendinitis. Working out too hard can cause fibers in your tendon to tear. And wearing the wrong type shoes can stretch your achilles tendon, leading to achilles tendinitis.

Tendon Connects muscle to bone.

Testosterone This is a male hormone. It stimulates bone and muscle growth and sexual development.

Thermogenesis Thermogenesis means increased fat loss by raising the body's core temperature. Or increased calorie burn as a result of a faster metabolism. Unfortunately, there are not a plethora of products on the market that can cause these changes to occur. More specifically, when this term is applied to B vitamins and popular herb products, it is probably a scam.

Thrombus This is a blood clot. It forms inside a blood vessel.

Throwing It is not a women's fault that she throws like a girl. An awkward looking overhand throw is not gender specific. It is all about training and experience. If you don't believe me, try throwing with your non-dominant arm.

Tibialis Anterior The muscle on the front of your shin.

Training Motivation Get a healthy perspective. Make friends with your body. It deserves your kindness. Then, make better choices. Walk away from sedentary life. Include more physical activity and healthier foods into your day. Soon you'll feel better both mentally and physically.

Trans Fatty Acid Usually found in margarine, this is a fatty acid that has been hydrogenated.

Transcutaneous Electrical Nerve Stimulation (TENS) Chiropractors use this modality to decrease pain in their patients. It provides a low-voltage electrical current

Transverse Abdominis Your transverse abdominis is beneath your obliques. It allows you to compress forcefully when you cough, sneeze, vomit, or use the restroom.

Trapezius These are the muscles on your upper shoulder beside your neck.

Triceps These are the muscles in the back of your upper arm.

Trigger Point A painful area to the touch, that when palpated, elicits pain elsewhere in your body. Locate a tender, nodular area within one of your muscles. This is called your trigger point. Gently massage it. Your goal is to restore normal, rich blood and oxygen flow to all parts your muscle. Trigger points strangulate areas of muscles, cutting off the normal nutrition and lifeline, compromising your muscles' function.

Triglycerides This is fat. It is made from three fatty-acid molecules and one glycerol molecule.

Trypsin An enzyme that is secreted by the pancreas. It helps you to digest proteins.

Ulcer An ulcer is an area of raw tissue, similar to the tissue found under the scab of a healing cut. Ulcers can occur in the stomach, or in the part of the intestine that drains food from the stomach.

Ulcerative Colitis A form of inflammatory bowel disease. The inner layer of your colon wall is damaged. Symptoms include abdominal pain, diarrhea, fever, weight loss, and blood in the stool.

Ultrasound An imaging technique used by doctors to view blood vessels and measure how fast blood is flowing. It uses high-frequency sound waves.

Ultrasound for Healing Exercise makes your bones stronger. And so does ultrasound. Ultrasound puts a soundwave into your bone which creates a pressure against the bone. This causes the same stress and strengthening that exercise does.

Unsaturated Fats Fatty acids in which some of the hydrogen atoms in each molecule have been replaced by double bonds (see polyunsaturated fats and monounsaturated fats).

Upper/Lower Body Exercises If you work your upper and lower body together as in a cross-country ski machine, your sympathetic nervous system kicks in, increasing your perceived exertion, making the exercise feel more difficult even though you may be burning the same amount of calories as doing a simple lower body cycling exercise.

Urethra This is a tube that transports urine from the bladder out of the body.

Varicose Veins Varicose veins affect more women then men, and the problem increases with age. A valve incompetency causes a reversal of blood flow. This dilates your veins and causes loss of tissue tone. There is a loss of elasticity in the walls of the affected veins and their valves. Because of their inefficiency, blood may stagnate in the vein. The veins become swollen and twisted. This may lead to fatigue and aching in the affected area.

Vein These are the vessels that carries blood back to your heart.

Vitamins Vitamins assist chemical reactions in your body. There are thirteen known vitamins. Four are fat-soluble— A, D, E, and K— which your body is able to store in amounts large enough to last for months. There are nine water-soluble vitamins— C (ascorbic acid), and the B-complex vitamins—B1 (thiamin), B2 (riboflavin), B6 (pyridoxine), B12, niacin, folic acid, biotin, and pantothenic acid. Your body needs replenishment of these vitamins regularly.

Warm-up Warm up before your martial arts training. Stretch afterwards. A warm up gives your joints a five to ten percent increase in synovial fluid. Stretch after your workout when your muscles are thoroughly heated up.

White-Coat Hypertension If you go to the doctor and your blood pressure is high, but when you take it at home it is normal, you might have white-coat hypertension.

Whooping Cough *Bordetella pertussis,* is the bacteria that causes whooping cough. It is transmitted from an infected person who coughed or sneezed in your direction *Pertussis* invades your respiratory mucosa causing increased secretion of mucus. At first it is a thin layer. Later it becomes viscous, and is not easily moved. Whooping cough lasts about six weeks.

Yeast Infections Most women get yeast infections at some time in their lives. A variety of microscopic organisms normally reside in the vagina. These include yeast-like fungus *Candida albicans.* But taking antibiotics can kill off certain flora and leave *Candida* to go on a rampage. This leads to Candida vaginitis, or a yeast infection.

Zone Diet A low carbohydrate, moderate protein, moderate fat diet in a ratio of forty percent carbohydrates, thirty percent protein, and thirty percent fat. It has not been shown to benefit long term weight loss.

Index

Books & Videos from YMAA

YMAA Publication Center Books

YMAA Publication Center Videotapes

YMAA Publication Center   楊氏東方文化出版中心

4354 Washington Street Roslindale, MA 02131
1-800-669-8892 • ymaa@aol.com • www.ymaa.com